Men's Health:
A Guide to
STAYING YOUNG

By the Editors of
Men's Health Magazine

MJF BOOKS
NEW YORK

Published by MJF Books
Fine Communications
Two Lincoln Square
60 West 66th St.
New York, NY 10023

Library of Congress Catalog Card Number 94-74189
ISBN 1-56731-069-9

Printed by arrangement with Rodale Press.

Men's Health is a registered trademark of Rodale Press, Inc.

This book was previously published by Rodale Press as *How a Man
Stays Young*.

Manufactured in the United States of America

MJF Books and the MJF colophon are trademarks of Fine Creative
Media, Inc.

10   9   8   7   6   5   4   3

Contributors

EXECUTIVE EDITOR, *Men's Health* magazine: Michael Lafavore

EDITORIAL DIRECTOR, *Men's Health* Books: Russell Wild

GROUP VICE-PRESIDENT: Mark Bricklin

PROJECT COORDINATOR: Dominick Bosco

BOOK DESIGNERS: Alfred Zelcer, Chuck Beasley

ILLUSTRATOR: Timothy Carroll

PRODUCTION EDITOR: Jane Sherman

COPY EDITOR: Rachelle Vander Schaaf

MANAGING EDITOR, *Men's Health* magazine: Steven Slon

RESEARCH EDITOR, *Men's Health* magazine: Melissa Gotthardt

OFFICE STAFF, *Men's Health* Books: Julie Kehs, Roberta Mulliner, Mary Lou Stephen

OFFICE MANAGER, *Men's Health* magazine: Susan Campbell

Contents

Introduction

GROPING FOR THE
FOUNTAIN OF YOUTH

The other day, a buddy of mine told me he's convinced that scientists will soon come up with a cure for aging. "Look," he argued, "technology is going crazy. They've got drugs to grow hair, lower cholesterol, prevent heart attacks and smooth out wrinkles. Don't tell me there aren't a bunch of researchers out there working on an anti-aging drug. It would be worth zillions."

When they start bottling eternal youth, I'll be the first in line to buy a six-pack. In the meantime, though, I'm not taking any chances. I've already started taking control of my own future. As noted health researcher Ben Douglas, Ph.D., tells us in chapter 1: "Many of the things that we blame on aging really have nothing to do with getting older." At 40, 50 or 60 years old, things like diminished vitality, strength and sexual vigor, mental fogginess, even most wrinkling, are not natural side effects of aging.

If you want to stay young longer, use this book as your guide. It will show you how to keep your body in shape, your nutrition up to peak levels, your stress under control, your relationships healthy and your sex life vital.

Another expert, Huber Warner, Ph.D., of the National Institute on Aging, tells us (in the same chapter): "The problems that lead to aging are cumulative, and the sooner you start correcting them, the better off you are in the long run." In other words, don't be like my friend and sit around waiting for someone to discover the Fountain of Youth. It's out there. Jump right in!

In addition to helping you stay young, this book will help you to boost your career, sharpen your image and get more fun out of life. Come to think of it, I'll have to pass a copy to my buddy!

Michael Lafavore
Executive Editor
Men's Health magazine

Part 1

HOW A MAN
STAYS YOUNG

Long-Distance Youth

Want to stay younger longer? Here's the
Men's Health *Look-Good, Feel-Great, Head-to-Toe,*
Anti-Aging Plan to tell you how to do it.

••••••••••••••••••••••

AGING HAS A WAY of leapfrogging up your list of concerns—from somewhere below "I'd better clean out those rain gutters soon" to "Alert! Alert! Top Priority! Code Red!"—in short order. The catalyst might be noticing a wrinkle that wasn't there the last time you looked, trying on a favorite shirt that's suddenly become too tight or playing a routine game of tennis and finding yourself creaky and sore afterward. One day you're thinking of yourself as a young man; the next day you're not so sure.

Fortunately, doctors and researchers are starting to pay as much attention to the subject of aging as the rest of us are. They're working to better understand the changes that come as we get older and what can be done about them. One thing is already clear from their studies: Aging is inevitable—there's no way to stop the clock—but a gradual decline in good health and good looks isn't.

"Many of the things we blame on aging really have nothing to do with getting older," says Ben Douglas, Ph.D., professor of anatomy at the University of Mississippi Medical Center and author of *AgeLess: Living Younger Longer*. He and others believe that we're genetically programmed to age at a certain rate but that most people are sapped of an extra measure of youth by diseases and a gradual buildup of preventable niggling insults to the body. As a rule, experts say, people could look younger, feel more vital and live much longer than they do.

"People should be concerned about aging from the earliest stages of their lives," says Huber Warner, Ph.D., of the National Institute on Aging (NIA). "The problems that lead to aging are cumulative, and the sooner you start correcting them, the better off you are in the long run. I've lived by that advice myself, and at age 55, my own experience tells me I feel better for it."

How can we stay young longer? *Men's Health* called on a wide-ranging field of experts on aging and the problems that attend it and asked them that question. This is the best of their advice.

GET PUMPING

A regular weight-training plan can make you feel—and look—decades younger. Recent research indicates that building muscle strength provides greater benefits to your health and vitality than was previously thought. Combined with a regimen of aerobic exercise, weight training strengthens your heart, boosts energy levels and protects you from injuries. It'll even improve your sex life, says Mark H. Cline, Ph.D., of the Male Health Center in Dallas. "When you're physically stronger, you're more robust, you have more energy and you're more likely to be sexually active."

Plus, it helps keep you looking great. Weight training shapes and tones muscles better than aerobic conditioning, and it wards off flab. "As a result, the average man who lifts weights will look even better than an endurance athlete when they're both older," says John Holloszy, M.D., a researcher at Washington University School of Medicine in St. Louis.

It's never too late to take up weight training. According to Tufts University researchers, even people in their nineties were able to increase their leg strength by as much as 200 percent by working out on weight-training equipment. It takes only one weight workout per week to maintain strength well into old age once you've made your initial gains (which takes about ten weeks of lifting two or three times a week).

TAKE ASPIRIN

Nothing on earth is more debilitating than being cut down in the prime of life by a stroke, the destruction of a portion of the brain caused by a blockage of blood flow to the area. Even a mild attack can leave a man temporarily paralyzed, blind or unable to talk. An estimated 300,000 men suffer strokes each year—and 100,000 will die, according to the National Stroke Association. Doctors say many of those tragedies could be prevented.

New studies show that taking regular doses of aspirin, especially if you have a history of heart or circulation problems, offers significant protection from strokes. Aspirin helps keep arteries from clogging up and blocking blood flow to the brain or heart.

It takes only small doses of aspirin to attain these benefits. "We're talking 30 to 81 milligrams," says New York physician Isadore Rossman, M.D., Ph.D., author of *Looking Forward: The Complete Medical Guide to Successful Aging.* Your pharmacist may stock 81-milligram doses, but if you can't find them, breaking a standard 325-milligram tablet into quarters will give you four correct doses. (Check with your doctor before starting an aspirin regimen.) How often you take aspirin is just as important as how much: Preventive effects are greatest when you take one 81-milligram dose every day or every other day.

In addition to protecting your heart, some studies suggest that taking aspirin regularly can reduce risk of colon cancer and cataracts, protect against gallstones and boost three important immune-system chemicals.

Since high blood pressure is a major cause of strokes, you can help protect yourself by getting your blood pressure checked as often as possible. A study found that systolic pressure (the top number) is a more accurate predictor of stroke risk than the diastolic reading (the bottom number).

CUT BACK ON PROTEIN

Your body needs protein for building everything from muscle to bone. Unfortunately, it doesn't need as much as most of us give it.

"The average American eats twice the protein he needs," says Art Mollen, D.O., medical director of the Southwest Health Institute in Phoenix and author of *The Anti-Aging Diet*. An excess of protein can make you feel heavy, sluggish and, over time, physically feeble. Dr. Mollen and others say we'd be better off eating more like the rural Chinese, whose grain-and-vegetable diet is extremely low in animal protein and whose death rate from colon cancer is about 2.5 times lower than ours.

For optimal health, eat 1 gram of protein for every 3 pounds of body weight per day, suggests Dr. Mollen. That's about 50 grams for a 150-pound man. A small portion of sirloin steak trimmed of fat contains about 35 grams, so limit yourself to one protein-based meal per day. "If you have a hamburger for lunch, that's fine, but have cereal or fruit for breakfast and pasta for dinner," says Dr. Mollen.

• •

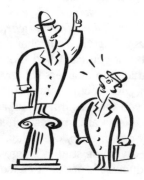

The Inner Winner
People who remember their strengths and successes more than their weaknesses and failures have what researchers at the University of California and Southern Methodist University call *positive illusions*. Such optimistic types are happier and work harder and longer—thus they often perform better.

DROP POUNDS, NOT CALORIES

We all want to cut a trim profile around the middle. A lean physique looks better, and more youthful, than a pear-shaped one. Lean men are also more active, more energetic and statistically less prone to chronic debilitating illnesses like diabetes and heart disease. To stay slim, however, men mistakenly tend to cut back on calories, when the real villain is lack of exercise and too much fat, says Eric Poehlman, Ph.D., a researcher of aging at the University of Vermont's Department of Medicine.

In fact, trying to keep weight off simply by cutting calories may not be a smart idea. By eating less, you risk cheating your body of important nutrients, says Dr. Poehlman. His formula for healthy weight loss is to exercise more as you reach middle age and to *eat more calories* as well. Just be sure they're low-fat calories. As a rule of thumb, 60 to 70 percent of your diet should consist of foods high in complex carbohydrates, such as bread, pasta and beans.

SUPPLEMENT YOUR DIET

You can protect yourself against both heart disease and cancer by getting more of the powerhouse vitamins E and C and the nutrient beta-carotene. All three can reduce your levels of free radicals, damaged molecules that cause harmful changes in the body. One theory holds that the aging process itself is the cumulative result of wear and tear from free radicals.

Unlike many other nutrients, vitamins E and C and beta-carotene are safe to take in amounts higher than the Recommended Dietary Allowance. "Since the risk is nil, it's safe to take more," says Jeffrey Blumberg, Ph.D., professor of nutrition at Tufts University. He suggests that optimal intakes for antioxidants may be in the range of 100 to 400 international units of vitamin E, 500 to 1,000 milligrams of vitamin C and 15 to 25 milligrams of beta-carotene every day.

HAVE PLENTY OF SEX

Physically, there's no getting around the fact that there's going to be some decrease in the pure animal drive you felt as a teenager. That's partly because, as you leave your teen years, you begin to have more to think about than sex. There is also some slowing down of the basic equipment as the arteries that carry blood to the penis lose flexibility. A regular exercise program can help remedy this by clearing away fatty deposits on arterial walls.

And, while there's no such thing as strength training for the penis, there is an exercise you can do to help keep your erections as firm as possible, says William Hartman, M.D., codirector of the Center for Marital and Sexual Studies in Long Beach, California. The exercise is often called a Kegel for men, and it works by strengthening the pelvic-floor muscles, the ones situated right beneath the base of the penis. First, find the right muscles: They're the ones you use to stop urine flow. Squeeze the muscles tightly for three seconds, then release. Start from a few and work up to 200 per day.

Just as important as keeping fit is continuing to have sex, not just for physical reasons, but for psychological ones as well. "Giving up on sex at any age can be symbolically giving up on all of life," says E. Douglas Whitehead, M.D., a New York urologist specializing in treating impotence. "It can drain vitality out of your marriage, your work, your sense of physical well-being and many of the other satisfactions that the second half of life can bring."

SHUN THE SUN

Yes, you've heard it. But if you're serious about keeping those youthful good looks of yours, you'd better *do* it. Sun damage is responsible for most of what we think of as aging. Skin damage builds up invisibly for years before you actually see it. In Australia, where men spend lots of time outdoors, scientists find sun damage causes wrinkling as early as age 20.

"The sun damages your skin completely," explains Karen Burke, M.D., of the Scripps Clinic and Research Foundation in La Jolla, California. "It gradually destroys your skin's inner elastic tissue and breaks down the connective tissue, all causing premature aging. As the outer layer of your skin thickens to protect the vital inner layers, your skin becomes leathery and old looking."

There's also new evidence that sunlight may play a role in the formation of gallstones. In a study, the risk of gallstones was 25 times greater for sunburn-prone subjects who sunbathed than for those who didn't. According to one theory, ultraviolet light from the sun, which triggers the skin's pigment system, may lead to an increase of pigments in the bile. This in turn could trigger gallstone formation.

No man is about to stay out of the sun altogether. But while you're out there, protect yourself by wearing a sunscreen with a sun protection factor (SPF) of 15 or higher, advises dermatologist Fredric Haberman, M.D., of Albert Einstein College of Medicine in New York City. "People think they need sunscreen only when they see the sun," Dr. Haberman says. "That's not true. You need it when it's cloudy, too, because clouds don't stop damaging ultraviolet rays." As added protection, he recommends wearing a hat with a brim to block damage from reflected light.

If you've already got wrinkles, you can do some repair work with Retin-A cream. Studies continue to show that regular use of this prescription medicine can eliminate the fine lines around the eyes and soften coarse wrinkles on the upper portions of the face. Dermatologists are now combining Retin-A with alpha hydroxy acids to reduce the irritation and redness that some people experience when they begin to use the medication.

STAND UP TO AGING

A hunched-over posture won't cause any medical problems, but it will certainly make you look old before your time. Most posture problems result from bad habits or weak back muscles. Start by fixing the habit: To walk tall, keep your rear tucked in, pull in your chin, tighten your stomach muscles and keep your knees unlocked. Then, if your back muscles are weak or frequently feel stiff, join a health club and ask your health instructor for specific exercises to correct the problem.

For the long term, you also need to guard your bones against loss of calcium. Men lose this mineral more slowly than women do, but we *do* lose it, especially in the spine, says Richard Sprott, Ph.D., who heads the NIA's Biology-of-Aging Program. Too little calcium can eventually make you slouch and can also lead to greater risk of crippling injury. To get enough, experts recommend eating calcium-rich foods such as skim milk, lowfat cheese, low-fat yogurt, broccoli, nuts and dried fruits. Also important is regular exercise, particularly weight training, which makes bones denser and stronger.

BOLSTER YOUR BACK

One minute you're zooming purposefully out the door on your way to hammer an opponent at racquetball; then you stoop for your gym bag and *boing,* you're instantly a crippled old man who can barely hobble to the nearest chair. "I've had back pain myself, and I can tell you that when you can barely move, and you can't play sports or exercise, it profoundly changes your life and your whole sense of well-being," says Alexis P. Shelekov, M.D., a spine surgeon at the Texas Back Institute in Dallas.

Most back troubles are minor problems caused by weak muscles, particularly the abdominals, which provide most of the spine's support. To strengthen them, Dr. Shelekov recommends walking, in conjunction with curl-ups: Lie on your back with your knees bent and your hands on your thighs. Keeping your lower back pressed to the ground, lift your head, neck and shoulders. Hold for a count of two; return. Start with five per day, working up to three sets of ten. As your abdominals become stronger, try the curl-ups with your hands across your chest.

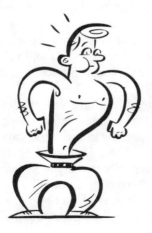

Age Eraser

Even if you don't exercise, breathing deeply can keep your lungs young, says Ken Douglas of the University of Mississippi. Inhale and exhale all the air you can, repeating several times. "If you do this every day and don't smoke, by age 70 you'll have the lungs of a 45-year-old," he says. As a result, you'll be less fatigued. "A lot of the tiredness we feel as we age is due to a decrease in oxygen to the body's systems," he says.

GET ENOUGH SLEEP

The legions of sleep-deprived stumble to their desks every morning, dragging themselves through the day fired with coffee and sugar and...excuse me, what were we talking about?

"Lack of rest at any age is going to make you *feel* old," says Michael Vitiello, associate director of the Sleep and Aging Research Program at the University of Washington in Seattle. Fatigue makes you physically slow and mentally dull. How much sleep is enough? "It's not so important how long you sleep as how good you feel during the day as a result," says Vitiello. "If you always feel draggy in the morning or late afternoon, you probably need more time in bed." To rest best, he advises turning in and getting up at the same times every day in order to keep your body clock in sync.

HAVE A DRINK

Research continues to pour in showing that moderate drinking (one or two alcoholic drinks per day—no more) protects against heart disease. In fact, drinking men in one recent study had less risk of death from heart disease than men who never touch the stuff.

Alcohol boosts levels of HDL cholesterol (the good kind), "and there are surprisingly few things that'll do that," says Dr. Rossman. Still, doctors are cautious about prescribing alcohol as preventive medicine, since heavy drinking damages the heart, brain and liver. Can you draw the line at a drink or two a day? If not, well, you're a big boy; you're better off saying no.

STIMULATE YOUR MIND

Your brain is not unlike your brawn. Exercise it and it'll get bigger and stronger. There's not much sense working to have the body of a 20-year-old if your mental capacity is slowly sliding toward senility.

Experts say mental challenges can sharpen your thinking. In one four-year study, healthy older people who stayed employed or did volunteer work or gardening had more blood flowing to their brains and did significantly better on IQ tests than their less active peers did. What's more, research suggests that people whose minds stay sharp into old age also live longer.

To keep your mind stimulated, indulge in hobbies and puzzles that are different from what you do on the job; they'll make your mind work in new ways (and have the added benefit of relaxing you). Socializing of any kind keeps the mind geared up for conversation. Reading a variety of newspapers gives you different perspectives on similar events.

You can also keep your mind fit by keeping your body fit. Long-term aerobic exercise has been shown to help keep older people mentally sharp, according to research at the Medical College of Pennsylvania. A study there found that men age 60 and older who had exercised regularly for five or more years scored significantly higher than nonexercisers of the same age on tests measuring mental quickness and recall.

LIVE WELL

Is aging a state of mind? There's not much science to prove it, but a surprising number of the researchers and doctors we spoke to said that you'll stay young if you think young. Among the benefits mentioned: A positive outlook will help you stick with an exercise program, take an interest in others and stay active longer.

A positive attitude is largely a matter of feeling you have control over your life, says Robin Barr, Ph.D., of the NIA's Adult Psychological Development Program. He points to studies of men in nursing homes who stay healthier and live longer solely by virtue of, for example, being free to find their own way to the lunchroom rather than being taken there.

"In the end, aging is a way of thinking," says Dr. Douglas. "In the past, we've thought that a person was old at age 65. It just isn't the case at all."

—Richard Laliberte

The Muscular Mind

It's not what you've got; it's how you use it. Here's a guide to maximizing your brain power—at any age.

●●●●●●●●●●●●●●●●●●●●●●●●

THE SUN WAS gleaming through clear Denver skies as United Airlines flight 232 bound for Chicago took off on the afternoon of July 19, 1989. All aboard expected a routine trip. And so it was, until 3:16 P.M., when the tail engine suddenly exploded. Passengers rocked forward and attendants plummeted to the floor as the huge DC-10 pitched downward.

With the two remaining jets under the wings, the plane still had power enough to fly. But power wasn't the problem. The blast had demolished the aircraft's hydraulic system, causing a complete loss of control of the rudder, wing flaps and ailerons. The 296 passengers were trapped at 37,000 feet in a plane with no steering. Captain Alfred C. Haynes had some fast thinking to do.

The situation called for an emergency landing, but the nearest strip was at Iowa's Sioux City Airport, 70 miles away. Although the steering was shot, Haynes found he could maintain some control by alternating speeds of the two wing jets. For 41 minutes, he and his three-man crew struggled to guide the disabled plane closer to the airport. On approach, Haynes shouted through the intercom, "Brace! Brace! Brace!" Moments later, the highly unstable aircraft somersaulted to the ground. Miraculously, 184 survived, many without a scratch.

For landing his plane against staggering odds, Haynes was commended for his exceptionally clear thinking and called a national hero, a label he had a hard time accepting. "There is no hero," he said. "There is just a group of four people, four people who did their job."

Perhaps, but by some standards Haynes is overly modest. "If you look at heroes in the movies, it's always the person who knows the right thing to do," says psychologist Dorothy Tennov, Ph.D. "Superman not only had great strength, he knew how to use it."

While most of the important decisions we make in life are made in less dramatic circumstances than Captain Haynes's, or Superman's for that matter, there are lessons for all of us here. The most important one is that no amount of training can compensate for crystal-clear thinking. Whether your decision concerns an investment, a job, a new house or which set of parents you're going to visit for Easter, clear thinking can help you make the best one.

Clear thinkers aren't born that way. They work at it. Before making important choices, they try to clear emotion, bias, trivia and preconceived notions out of the way so they can concentrate on the information essential to making the right decision.

If your thinking isn't always as focused as you'd like it to be or if you find that you often make choices you later regret, especially if you have to make them quickly, it's time for a course in clear thinking. Here are a few lessons from some of the best-known people in the business.

ASSEMBLE THE FACTS

Before you can make a good decision, you have to assemble all the facts—not just the obvious stuff, but everything you can get your hands on. Although Captain Haynes's time was extremely limited, he had to gather certain information before he could choose a course of action. How much damage had the explosion caused? Which controls were still available to him? What sites were open for an emergency landing?

"Mistakes are usually made because someone had insufficient or bad data," says John C. Johnson, M.D., director of emergency medical services at Porter Memorial Hospital in Valparaiso, Indiana.

The way to get good data is to ask questions. At the emergency room, Dr. Johnson is faced with life-or-death crises daily. His powers of observation and a willingness to think beyond the obvious are what get him through. For example, he describes the case of a badly wheezing child whisked into the emergency room for care. If the attending doctor wasn't thinking clearly, he might reason that the child was having an asthma attack and treat him accordingly. But a sharper doctor would first ascertain when the wheezing began and whether the child had been playing with any small objects. He might discover that the child was choking—and save a life.

As Sherlock Holmes said to the ever-bumbling Watson: "It is a capital mistake to theorize before you have all the evidence. It biases the judgment."

LOOK UNDER EVERY ROCK
FOR HIDDEN OPPORTUNITIES

Take the job/don't take the job. Can't decide? What about other choices? In just about any given situation, a little thinking turns up more options you could take. But if you're like most, you never seek out all those choices. It's easy to get forced into anxiety-ridden "either/or" situations.

One way you may be limiting your options is by springing upon the first solution to a problem that shows itself. But "your first answer is likely not to be your best," says Jeff Salzman, vice-president of CareerTrack, a Colorado-based consulting company. Instead say, "Okay, I have one possible answer—let's see if I can find something better."

The cerebral world of chess offers a perfect example of the importance of creative thinking. According to Michael Valvo, one of America's top-rated chess players, the downfall of many in chess—as in life—is that they "concentrate on only two or three moves, while at least seven or eight are usually available."

KEEP YOUR COOL

Imagine what was going through Captain Haynes's mind when he found himself in the cockpit of a crippled plane with the lives of nearly 300 people depending on his judgment. Did he wring his hands? Did he visualize the flaming destruction that could have been moments away?

Of course not. If he had, there'd be no story to tell. "I really didn't have any thoughts," he says. "There was nothing on my mind but what we were trying to accomplish, just the job at hand, which was to bring the plane down safely."

How can you always be coolheaded, especially at a trying moment? The key, our experts agree, is self-confidence.

We know what you're probably thinking: *Easy for us to say.* Sure, Captain Haynes had confidence in his flying skills, but what about decisions that involve whole new sets of parameters you're not familiar with? Having self-confidence can be hard when you lack experience, agrees Dr. Johnson. His advice to young doctors who get hung up trying to decide if they're doing the right thing is to look to the good decisions they have made in the past to reinforce their confidence. There's no reason you can't do the same.

The heart of this issue is trust...of yourself. It's an attitude that has at its core an acceptance of yourself and your decisions regardless of what anybody else thinks or any mistakes you may have made, says Albert Ellis, Ph.D., president of the Institute for Rational Emotive Therapy in New York City.

BE AN "AMIABLE SKEPTIC"

The tough part about separating your emotions from your reasoning is that there are lots of people out there who'd rather you remain emotional—like the boss or spouse who uses emotion-inciting ploys to get you to do something you don't want to do. To prevent yourself from being lured into making bad decisions, it's important to view things with a critical eye, says Diane Halpern, Ph.D., a professor of psychology at California State University. That means developing what she calls an attitude of amiable skepticism. Amiable, because it doesn't entail an adversarial relationship with the world. You can be doubtful and still be cheerful. You can decide to reserve judgment when you sense you're being swayed against your will. It begins with advertising and extends to telephone salesmen offering trips to Hawaii for $300 and all the way to politicians promising to be kinder while they're acting tougher.

CREATE A BALANCE SHEET

Whatever decision is looming before you, you want to make the best one. You've already gathered all the information and searched hard to come up with many different avenues. Now it's rating time.

The best way to do it, say the experts, is to grab paper and pen and put together a list of all of the advantages and disadvantages of each option. You can use any rating system you like, but we favor the basic 1-to-10.

Then do some quick arithmetic. "You'll normally find that one option comes out with a distinctly better score," says Dr. Ellis. If you *don't* make such a list, he warns, you risk allowing your emotions to give a disproportionate weight to a single aspect.

He gives as an example a young man he knows who purchased a flashy—but quite undependable—car simply because it turbocharged his ego. Naturally, the guy soon found himself with a car he was kicking more than driving.

DROP YOUR "MUSTS"

While in the midst of trying to make a decision, any decision, listen to your inner self. Do you hear a cranky little voice inside saying, "I must have this…I must…I must…I *must!*" People are born with a tendency to take their important desires and turn them into "musts," says Dr. Ellis.

The problem is that this limits your ability to think in an objective manner. The key to rational thinking and clear decision-making is to remain flexible. So the next time you hear yourself saying "I *must!*" step back and ask yourself, "*Must* I?" Ask yourself if the sabbatical you've been fantasizing about taking really makes more sense after the kids get out of college; consider whether a dependable car might make more sense than that Porsche 911 you saw in the used-car lot. You might be surprised how good it feels to make the more logical (read: grown-up) choice.

CHOP UP BIG DECISIONS

A big decision can be like an enormous chunk of steak. Try to swallow it without first cutting it up, and you risk choking. So says Paul Slovic, Ph.D., professor of psychology at the University of Oregon and president of Decision Research, a nonprofit research institute in Eugene, who recommends a technique he calls "incrementalism." Say, for instance, that you're considering giving up your job as a salesman in Chicago to become a sportswriter in Miami. The decision involves not only starting a new career but selling your house, moving your family and leaving all your friends. You've been agonizing over this one for some time.

Decisions like this can be overwhelming, says Dr. Slovic. The thing to do if you feel overwhelmed is to cut up the dilemma into smaller pieces. Perhaps you can find a part-time newspaper job in Chicago, while keeping your present job, to see if reporting will be as much to your liking as you think. Possibly you can take time off from work and spend it in Miami with the family to see how much everyone goes for Florida living. You may be surprised. "We tend to think that we can predict new situations better than we actually can," says Dr. Slovic.

GET A SECOND OPINION

When time allows, it's a good idea to consult with other people before making important decisions. There are just too many things in this world that are too big for any one person to examine alone.

But whose opinion do you ask? You could go to your best friend or someone else with whom you share common interests and values. But you'll do much better by asking people who think differently. People who are like you will probably agree with you. That will boost your confidence, but not the accuracy of the decision.

A better tactic is to go to people with different backgrounds, different occupations—different biases. And if you want to get double your money's worth from a second opinion, ask for it before you reveal your own feelings, say the experts. Don't walk in and say, "I've decided that I'm going to get this operation—what do *you* think?" The advice you get will be much more valuable if it comes without any influence from you.

DON'T RUSH THE VERDICT

The old advice "Sleep on it" makes a lot of sense. Your opinions will be more valuable if you harvest them after allowing them time to ripen. Your vision becomes clearer over time about decisions and judgments you need to make.

There's a good reason for this. "We're heavily influenced by recency," says Donald A. Norman, Ph.D., a professor of cognitive science at the University of California in San Diego.

For instance, if you had to travel to London two days after a major airline crash, you might seriously think about canceling the trip. "Leaving a little time to put recent things in the past can help a lot to clarify thinking," he says.

PROVE YOURSELF WRONG

Most of us, when we make up our minds, set out immediately to validate what we think we "know," says Dr. Ellis. As time goes on, we find more and more "proof" that our assumptions are correct because all we're looking for is that proof. "But we tend to learn more by trying to falsify our assumptions," says Dr. Ellis.

There's no better way to find holes in the fabric of faulty thinking than to ask yourself, "What are the reasons I may be wrong?" Try asking this question of yourself the next time you feel absolutely sure about something. You've got nothing to lose but your possible error!

—Russell Wild

Take Two Risks and Call Me in the Morning

There's nothing more empowering for a man than to meet his fears and overcome them. So take some risks now and then. The doctor says it will be good for you.

••••••••••••••••••••••

BY MOST ACCOUNTS, my college roommate was a conservative fellow. He voted for Reagan, preferred playing the piano to partying and was usually asleep by 11:00 P.M. He appeared to be the embodiment of dullness and predictability. But one Saturday morning, while I was still in bed trying to determine the molecular weight of a can of Budweiser, he burst into the room with a smug grin on his face. "I just jumped out of a plane at 10,000 feet," he said. "I'm going to do it again tomorrow. Wanna try it?"

I politely declined. I've never been that crazy about the idea of riding in airplanes, let alone leaping out of them. What if the guy who packed my parachute had a really bad hangover that day? What if I drifted into a high-tension power line and got roasted? What if I landed in the lagoon of a sewage-treatment plant and drowned? Hadn't I read about that happening to someone a few years ago?

I think I know why my buddy did something so seemingly uncharacteristic, perhaps even foolhardy. He did it *because* it was uncharacteristic and foolhardy. He needed to travel to the edge and dance on it for a while because his life was so otherwise boring and predictable.

Everyone needs some of that risk and excitement. After all, in terms of evolution, we've been wearing suits and living in split-levels for only a speck of time. Most of our prehistoric past was filled with uncertainty, danger and extreme risks. The people who survived were those who thrived on those risks. We're their heirs, and that need for a certain amount of risk is still strong in us.

I don't need airplanes and parachutes to fulfill my adventure quotient; roller coasters do it for me. I get sweaty palms and a flip-flopping stomach just waiting in line. Being strapped in the seat is exquisite agony. By the time I reach the top of the first steep rise, I'm convinced that death is moments away. My heart is in my mouth through the entire ride. When it's over, I feel…terrific. I've spit in the eye of fear, grabbed myself an energizing jolt of adrenaline.

RISK BUILDS CHARACTER

Not only is this fun, it's good for me. Experts who have studied risk taking say it develops character and courage, extends creativity, boosts confidence and helps establish a sense of limitations and possibilities. They say that if you don't allow yourself some conscious risks, you may be more likely to take unconscious ones such as driving too fast, drinking too much, picking fights or gambling away money, relationships or a job.

"It's important to take risks to experience life," says Frank Farley, Ph.D., a psychologist at the University of Wisconsin. "If you don't expose yourself to new experiences and new ideas, you remain the same. And change is a very important part of personal growth."

Dr. Farley, who coined the term *T-Type personality* to describe people who love risks, says you don't have to run out and sign up for a course in rattlesnake wrestling to get a charge. "Anytime you can overcome a fear or meet a challenge and not run from it, it strengthens you as a person," he says. Dr. Farley considers healthy risk taking to be anything to which the outcome is uncertain. This includes not only obvious stuff like bungee jumping and rock climbing but also psychological and financial risks like starting a business, investing in the stock market or changing careers.

In fact, only the risk taker himself can determine what's risky. Some of us choose to take risks in one part of our lives but not in another. The defining element is fear. There's no thrill—and no real risk—without that. When Phillipe Petit, the acrobat who walked a wire between the World Trade Center towers, was asked about his feat, he said that balancing 110 stories above ground without a net wasn't all that scary for him.

What did he consider risky?

Spiders, snakes...and getting married, he replied. He'd rather do 10,000 backward somersaults on a high wire than get married and have kids.

FEAR OF FAILING

Fear is what makes us avoid risk, run away from challenges, play it safe. We do it to spare ourselves failure, embarrassment, bankruptcy, injury or death. But, says Dr. Farley, "There's nothing more empowering for a man than to meet his fears and overcome them." His studies show that risk takers are more self-confident, energetic, creative and independent than less daring men.

In nearly every high-risk sport, the mastery of fear comes up repeatedly as the principal reward for engaging in it. The deeper the fear, the bigger the thrill when you conquer it. One study found that the more frightened sky divers were while going up in a plane, the more exhilarated they felt when they parachuted safely to the ground.

According to Ralph Keyes, author of the book *Chancing It: Why We Take Risks,* that rush is delivered by natural opiate-like body chemicals that kick in during a stressful experience. "It's nature's way of rewarding us for taking chances," he says.

Keyes, who interviewed nearly a thousand T-Types for his book, says some people become addicted to that chemical kick and look for ever-more-challenging ways to keep it coming. A predisposition to thrill seeking, he adds, may even be genetic.

THE FOREIGN LEGION?

So maybe you're the kind of guy who likes to avoid the unexpected. You always keep a spare car key in a magnetic case under your bumper. You never leave the house without an umbrella. You wouldn't dream of tearing the label off a mattress. You know you're stuck in an unexciting rut, but you don't know what to do about it. Should you take up hang gliding? Plan a scuba trip to the shark feeding grounds off the Great Barrier Reef?

Probably not, says Dr. Farley. "Many men dream of breaking out of their everyday roles and becoming super-risk-taking heroes overnight, but it doesn't happen very often," he says. "You change by taking small steps into the unknown."

He suggests starting with minor changes. Identify some of your long-held fears and begin pushing them. If you're a creature of habit who always eats at the same restaurants,

• •

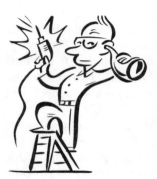

Age Eraser

To keep your hearing keen, wear ear protectors when operating mowers and other power equipment, and keep personal stereos turned down. (Some units can damage hearing at two-thirds volume.) Maintaining a low-fat diet and exercising can prevent atherosclerosis, which can gradually cause hearing loss.

make it a point to try some new ones. Instead of going on your usual vacation, ask your travel agent about adventure packages. Add variety to your sex life by experimenting with new places and positions. If you can't face a fear head on, try taking risks in another part of your life. "I've always wanted to be a stand-up comic, but I could never get up the nerve," admits Keyes. "Instead I went rock climbing and risked my neck. It was scary, but I was less frightened of that than of getting booed off a stage."

Given the lack of objective standards, how do you decide if a risk is worth taking? Ask yourself what you have to gain if you're successful and what you have to lose if you're not. Dabbling in the stock market is an acceptable risk if you have a few spare dollars; learning to drive a race car with a certified instructor is more likely to thrill you than kill you. On the other hand, going for a spin in your Delta 88 when you've got a bellyful of wine is just dangerous and stupid. (Dr. Farley calls drinking and driving and other purely reckless behaviors T-negative.)

What if you take a risk and fail? Big deal. According to Keyes, the biggest losers are those who never took risks in the first place. He tells of a sky diver who spent a year in the hospital after falling 2,000 feet when his chute failed to open. "Sure, he regretted the accident, but he didn't regret skydiving, and he was ready to go up again." Likewise, people who start businesses that fail, audition for parts they don't get or become deeply involved in relationships that don't pan out are usually proud of themselves for making the effort. "There's a sense of satisfaction in taking a risk—win or lose—that can't be found any other way," Keyes says. "People who choose *not* to take important risks often have deep regrets, almost to the point of mourning."

—*Dan Bensimhon*

(To measure your risk quotient, take the quiz beginning on page 22.)

· ·

HOW GUTSY ARE YOU

Are you an adventure-loving kind of guy, or is your idea of a big risk not guaranteeing a hotel room for late arrival? Is there a thrill seeker hidden inside that buttoned-down exterior of yours? Take this quiz to see if you're a Milquetoast or a maniac.

There are no right or wrong answers here, nor is any score better than another. Circle only one letter per question. Answer all questions. If no answer feels exactly right to you, pick the one that's closest. Then see "Scoring," on page 25.

1. During the past ten years, how often have you changed residence?
    a. 10 times or more
    b. 5–9 times
    c. 2–4 times
    d. 0–1 times

2. Which adjective best describes your behavior before age 12?
    a. hyperactive
    b. mischievous
    c. basically well behaved
    d. very well behaved

3. In an average week, how many hours of TV do you watch?
    a. 0–5
    b. 6–10
    c. 11–20
    d. more than 20

4. How often do you tape shut already-sealed envelopes before mailing them?
    a. almost never
    b. seldom
    c. often
    d. regularly

· ·

5. When eating Chinese food, how often do you use chopsticks?
- **a.** regularly
- **b.** often
- **c.** seldom
- **(d.)** almost never

6. On highways, how often do you drive faster than 65 mph?
- **a.** regularly
- **(b.)** often
- **c.** seldom
- **d.** almost never

7. If you were living on the East Coast a century ago, do you think you would have joined a wagon train headed west?
- **(a.)** definitely
- **b.** probably
- **c.** probably not
- **d.** definitely not

8. Suppose you had equal competence at any one of the following activities. Which would appeal to you most?
- **a.** skydiving
- **(b.)** mountain climbing
- **c.** producing a play
- **d.** building a house

Assume that you are equally skilled in all of the activities listed below. For each set, pick the one that you would most enjoy. (If neither activity appeals to you, pick the one that's least unappealing.)

9.
- **a.** driving a dune buggy
- **(b.)** hiking in the desert

(continued)

• •

HOW GUTSY ARE YOU—CONTINUED

10. **(a.)** skiing down a steep slope
   b. ski touring through woods

11. **(a.)** scuba diving
   b. snorkeling

Circle the letter for the word that best describes your reaction to the following activities.

12. Building a cabinet
   a. tedious
   (b.) satisfying

13. Climbing rocks
   (a.) exhilarating
   b. scary

14. Attending a rock concert
   (a.) arousing
   b. jarring

15. Teaching school
   a. boring
   (b.) challenging

16. With a report due at work in two weeks, you would be most likely to:
   a. start working on it the day before it's due, then stay up most of the night completing it
   (b.) work hard on the report for a day or two before it's due
   c. start working on it during the second week
   d. budget time throughout the two weeks to produce the report

• •

17. In general, you prefer the company of:
    a. people you've recently met
    b. professional colleagues, co-workers or fellow members of a club or church

18. Which opportunity sounds more appealing to you?
    a. starting your own business
    b. purchasing a successful business

19. Which statement describes you better?
    a. I get bored easily
    b. When necessary, I can tolerate routine

20. What kinds of risks would you say are hardest for you to take?
    a. commitment risks (ones involving long-term involvement with a person, faith, activity or career)
    b. emotional risks (in relationships, or showing my feelings)
    c. financial risks (of losing money)
    d. physical risks (of life and limb)

Scoring: Give yourself one point for each "a," two points for each "b," three for each "c" and four for each "d."

30 or below: Suggests a high need for excitement and a low tolerance for boredom. You're more likely than other men to take physical risks and to avoid emotional or long-term commitments. You're best suited to jobs that involve constant crises, such as emergency-room doctor, commodities trader or small-business owner. Potential problems: reckless driving, drug and alcohol abuse, compulsive gambling.

31 and above: Suggests you find it hard to take physical and financial risks but easy to take long-term risks, such as deciding to raise a family or committing yourself to a career. Tolerance for routine and ability to take the long view make you ideal for management or supervisory jobs. Potential problems: lethargy and depression.

Part 2

HEALTHY EATS

Nine Nutrients for Men

Men need more of just about every essential nutrient than women. Here are the nine most important vitamins and minerals that every man should know about.

• •

WHICH VITAMINS DO you need most, and how much do you need? *Men's Health* went to the experts for the answers. But first, an interesting footnote: Men and women have differing nutritional needs. In fact, the U.S. Food and Drug Administration puts out separate men's and women's lists of Recommended Dietary Allowances (RDA) for vitamins and minerals. And men need more of just about every essential nutrient than women do. Why? Quite simply, because we're bigger. We have more muscle and burn more calories than women do. And those of us who are fit and active, in particular, need higher quantities of certain key nutrients.

Further, getting enough of the right vitamins and minerals can help us fight problems we men are at especially high risk for, such as elevated cholesterol, hypertension, coronary heart disease, stroke, certain cancers and kidney stones.

Here, in alphabetical order, are the nine nutrients men need most.

CHROMIUM

This vital mineral can cut cholesterol, boost endurance in athletes and help bodybuilders gain muscle and lose fat. The average man needs at least 50 micrograms of chromium a day, but active men should get 100 to 200 micrograms, according to Richard Anderson, Ph.D., of the U.S. Department of Agriculture Human Nutrition Research Center. "You'll have a hard time getting this much from foods," he says. Your best source is a multivitamin/mineral complex that includes chromium. Next best is one or two chromium-fortified tablets of brewer's yeast daily.

FIBER

Technically, fiber's not a nutrient, since it passes through the body undigested. But eating fiber substantially reduces cholesterol and may help lower blood pressure. A high-fiber diet may lower your risk of colon cancer (the third most common kind for men) and can control sugar levels in diabetics. Fiber may even help you lose weight by filling you up without a lot of calories. Two medium-sized apples will give you 14 of the recommended 18 to 35 daily grams of dietary fiber you need. You also get fiber from whole-grain breads and breakfast cereals, brown rice, strawberries, pears and vegetables, especially ones with edible stalks and stems such as broccoli and carrots.

MAGNESIUM

This mineral plays a key role in regulating the heartbeat—studies show that getting enough may protect men against heart disease as well as bring down high blood pressure. Magnesium also boosts fertility by making sperm more vigorous. You'll get about two-thirds of your daily requirement of magnesium from a breakfast of two cups of shredded wheat, skim milk and a banana. Baked potatoes, beans, nuts, oatmeal, peanut butter, whole-wheat spaghetti, leafy vegetables and seafood are also magnesium rich.

VITAMIN A

Studies find vitamin A can have significant immunity-boosting and anticancer effects. And, yes, just as your mother told you, it helps maintain good vision. A ½-cup serving of steamed carrots supplies almost four times a man's daily recommended intake of 1,000 milligrams. Other good sources are liver, dairy products, fish, tomatoes, apricots and cantaloupe. Vitamin A is easy to get from your diet and extremely toxic in high doses, so experts recommend avoiding supplements.

VITAMIN B$_6$

This necessary nutrient is a powerful immune booster, and some studies suggest it may prevent skin and bladder cancer. Additionally, B$_6$ protects against the formation of kidney stones (a problem that afflicts twice as many men as women) and can help prevent restless sleep. You need only two milligrams of vitamin B$_6$ daily—about the amount in two large bananas. Active men need a few milligrams more, since it's burned up during exercise, says Paula Trumbo, Ph.D., assistant professor of nutritional biochemistry at Purdue University. Other dietary sources include chicken and fish, liver, potatoes, avocados and sunflower seeds. High doses of B$_6$ supplements can be toxic over time, so experts recommend taking no more than 50 milligrams a day.

VITAMIN C

It boosts immunity; may help prevent cancer, heart disease and stroke; promotes healthy gums and teeth; prevents cataracts; hastens wound healing; counteracts asthma; and may help overcome infertility in men. Keeping your body well supplied with vitamin C may also slow the aging process. Broccoli, cantaloupe, green peppers and grapefruit juice are good dietary sources, but supplements won't harm you, as this vitamin's not toxic in high doses. Researcher Earl Dawson, Ph.D., of the University of Texas Medical Branch, says 200 to 300 milligrams a day should be adequate. Many researchers think you'll shortchange yourself on vitamin C with the RDA of 60 milligrams (the amount in ½ cup of fresh orange juice), particularly when it comes to warding off the common cold, the most well known of C's benefits.

If you smoke, you probably need extra vitamin C. Smokers have lower levels of the vitamin in their blood. No one knows why, but the implication is that their bodies need more C and thus are using more.

VITAMIN E

Studies show vitamin E lowers cholesterol, prevents buildup of artery-clogging plaque, boosts immunity, cleanses the body of pollutants and prevents cataracts. There's lots of vitamin E in almonds, peanuts and pecans, but it's hard to get enough of this nutrient from your diet. Fortunately, supplements are safe in doses much higher than the 10-milligram RDA. Biochemist Max Horwitt, Ph.D., of the St. Louis University School of Medicine, takes 269 milligrams daily and considers that amount safe.

WATER

It's the most essential of all nutrients, especially if you're muscular: Muscle contains almost three times more water than fat. (The average man's body is 40 percent muscle, while the average woman's is 23 percent.) Water lubricates joints, regulates temperature and provides the body with minerals and essential fluids. The average man should get at least two quarts a day, or about eight glasses. "If you're physically active, you could easily need to double that," says Georgia Kostas, a registered dietitian and director of nutrition at the Cooper Clinic. You also get water from food: Bread is about 36 percent water; a potato, 80 percent.

ZINC

Getting enough zinc ensures that your sex drive, potency and fertility stay in shape. Zinc's been used experimentally to treat impotence, and it has a profound influence on the body's ability to heal wounds and resist disease. Men tend to get only about two-thirds the RDA of 15 milligrams, particularly if we're active. That's because when men sweat, we lose more zinc than women. One four-ounce helping of lean beef provides almost half the daily zinc needs. Other good sources are turkey, seafood, cereals and beans. Too much zinc can hinder the work of other minerals, so experts recommend taking no more than one 15-milligram supplement a day.

—Richard Laliberte

Designated Eaters

Looking for healthful substitutes for high-fat, high-calorie and low-fiber foods? Here are some smart swaps to get you on the healthy track.

••••••••••••••••••••••••

WHEN IT COMES TO EATING healthier, our motto is "Switch, don't fight." Don't do battle with your urges for satisfying foods in a quest for less fat and calories and more fiber; just switch to equally satisfying but more healthful alternatives.

An example: On the gratification scale, a roast beef sandwich with cheese comes close to a large cheeseburger, but the roast beef contains 43 percent less fat and 101 fewer calories. Not a bad deal.

If you find that one of these swaps doesn't immediately ring the same bells as its less healthy cousin, give it another chance. It often takes a little time for your brain's "pleasure centers" to adapt to something slightly different.

•••

Instead of . . .	Try . . .	Benefit
Salted peanuts	Pretzels	91% less fat
Potato chips	Popcorn, air-popped	96% less fat
Saltines	Animal crackers	22% less fat
Chocolate chip cookies	Fig bars	80% less fat
Caramels	Raisins	96% less fat
Pecan pie	Chocolate cake w/icing	32% less fat
Chocolate cake w/icing	Apple pie	28% less fat
Eclairs w/custard filling and chocolate icing	Angel food cake w/chocolate syrup	96% less fat
Glazed doughnuts	Blueberry muffins	59% less fat
Granola cereal	Raisin bran	89% less fat

(continued)

•••

Instead of . . .	Try . . .	Benefit
Peanut butter on bagel	Strawberry jam on bagel	99% less fat
Italian roll	Whole-wheat bread	87% more fiber
Regular mayonnaise on burger	Barbecue sauce on burger	84% less fat
Large cheeseburger	Roast beef sandwich w/cheese	101 fewer calories
Beef bologna	Turkey bologna	47% less fat
Sandwich w/cold cuts	Sandwich w/roast beef	27% less fat
Pepperoni pizza	Cheese pizza	48% less fat
Bean-and-meat burrito	Bean burrito	19% less fat
Macaroni and cheese	Spaghetti in tomato sauce w/cheese	170 fewer cal./cup
Prime rib, roasted	Sirloin, broiled	67% less fat
Chicken drumsticks, roasted	Chicken breasts, roasted	30% less fat
Steamed salmon	Baked cod	89% less fat
Lamb shoulder	Leg of lamb	28% less fat
Chocolate milk, whole	Chocolate milk, 1%	71% less fat
Half-and-half in coffee	Condensed skim milk in coffee	98% less fat

Note: Except where indicated, this chart compares 100-gram portions of each food.

—*Mary Brophy*

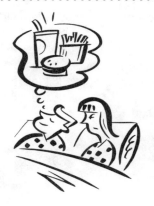

Junk Food Starves Your Sex Life

A steady diet of burgers, fries and other fatty foods could leave you sex-starved. A study at the University of Utah suggests that fat-laden meals may curb the production of testosterone, a hormone that fuels your sex drive.

Power Eating

We asked the medical experts to design an eating plan for total health. They came up with a dozen steps to peak nutrition.

• •

THERE IS CERTAINLY no shortage of self-proclaimed nutrition "experts" out there, from fitness gurus who make millions selling worthless supplement powders and pills to next-door neighbors who claim that eating white bread will send you to an early grave.

Who has the time to weigh all the contradictory advice, much less judge the validity of its source? Not you. And anyway, that's why you read books like this one.

To get straight answers for our readers, *Men's Health* surveyed 300 of the nation's top nutrition experts—not the self-appointed kind, but the ones doing important research at major hospitals and universities. Medical Consensus Surveys, a research arm of Rodale Press, asked the experts to rate 44 nutritional actions (all purported to benefit health) as follows: Extremely Important, Very Important, Important, Not Important or Probably Worthless.

What we were after was a list of priorities, a simple guide to making smart nutritional choices. For example, should you put a lot of energy into reducing the amount of cholesterol in your diet? The amount of salt? Or is it more important to avoid pesticides, irradiated food or alcohol?

The nutritionists' responses were then compiled and statistically weighted to create a list of dietary priorities that's both clear and practical. "We could easily have an enormous advance in the health of America if we could simply follow these guidelines," says George L. Blackburn, M.D., Ph.D., chief of the Nutrition/Metabolism Laboratory at New England Deaconess Hospital in Boston.

Here, in order of importance, are the nutritional steps most vital to your healthy diet and the stuff that's not worth worrying about.

GET THE FAT OUT

The experts were almost unanimous in putting weight control at the top of the list—97 percent of them gave it high priority.

"If everybody in the United States maintained their ideal weight, the incidence of Type-II diabetes would be greatly reduced, hypertension would be much less common and so would coronary disease," says Meir Stampfer, M.D., associate professor of epidemiology at Harvard School of Public Health.

Nearly 24 percent of American men are overweight for their age and build, which makes obesity one of the country's biggest health problems.

How do the experts recommend we lose weight? Seventy-five percent said that cutting calories is Extremely Important or Very Important; 70 percent said the same about controlling fat intake. The two go hand in hand: If you cut calories, you'll cut fat. The number of calories you eat ultimately determines how much you'll weigh, but reducing fat is important for other reasons: It slashes the risk of heart disease by keeping arteries from choking with plaque, and it may reduce the risk of some forms of cancer.

EAT AND RUN

Strictly speaking, exercise isn't a nutritional habit, but we included it in our survey because physical activity has a direct bearing on how much we eat and what happens to food once we've taken it in. The experts affirmed this view, and then some. Eighty-four percent gave high priority to exercising more. "It's hard to reduce your weight by controlling calories alone," says Dr. Stampfer. "If you exercise as well, you're more likely to be able to maintain the weight loss in the long run."

Exercise boosts your metabolism, allowing you to eat more without putting on more pounds. It also helps relieve stress and keep your heart, bones and circulatory system in top form.

Most people can fill their exercise quota with 20 minutes of brisk walking three times a week. Adding a regimen of resistance weight training fires up your metabolism to its calorie-burning peak.

DON'T LIKE IT, DON'T EAT IT

Giving up all your favorite foods and switching to a very healthy but very boring diet won't work. Kelly Brownell, Ph.D., professor of psychology at Yale University and a top obesity researcher, says he and others have studied dieters and found that the most punishing methods inevitably fail.

Nobody is going to eat food they don't enjoy for very long. If you want to eat healthy, you have to either find low-fat prepared foods that taste great or learn to cook your own.

KEEP IT BALANCED BUT LEAN

You've heard the old nutritionists' creed: Balance your diet among the four food groups, and make sure you get the Recommended Dietary Allowance (RDA) of vitamins and minerals. These concepts are certainly not passé; roughly 90 percent of those surveyed said they're still high priority. Yet those notions now clearly take a backseat to cutting fat and controlling weight.

The weakness of the four-food-groups approach is that it doesn't provide enough guidance to prevent you from eating too much fat and amassing too much of it on your body.

If you make fat-fighting your number one priority, however, it quite naturally leads you toward fulfilling those other guidelines. "If you phase out the high-calorie, high-fat foods in your diet, you're going to have to replace them with something low-fat—cereals, fruits and vegetables," says Dr. Blackburn. An emphasis on those foods moves you closer to meeting your RDA for vitamins and minerals. It can also move you closer to balancing your diet, which for most Americans is overladen with high-fat meat and dairy products.

DON'T SWEAT THE TECHNICALITIES

If you've never been able to keep straight the difference between saturated, unsaturated, monounsaturated and polyunsaturated fats, here's good news: You don't have to. The trendy notion that you should trade saturated fats for heart-smarter monounsaturated and polyunsaturated ones is "putting the cart before the horse," according to Dr. Blackburn. Most of the foods that are highest in total fat—ice cream, cheeseburgers and doughnuts, for example—are also highest in saturated fat. So if you simply cut down on all fatty foods, you'll cut down on saturated fat as well.

How much fat should you eat? The nutritionists advise following the American Heart Association's recommendation that total dietary fat comprise no more than 30 percent of calories.

LET CHOLESTEROL TAKE CARE OF ITSELF

Cutting cholesterol scored surprisingly low. Only 14 percent of the experts rated it Extremely Important. It's not that cholesterol is insignificant, but, again, if you follow the priorities outlined above, you'll have already taken care of it. Those polled felt that excessive concern about this issue to the exclusion of all others could lead you to eat foods that are low in cholesterol but still dangerously high in fat. For example, potato chips fried in vegetable oil contain no cholesterol, but 72 percent of their calories are from fat.

DON'T FEAR SAYING "CHEERS"

The nation's top nutritionists plainly don't support prohibition. But they're staunch believers in moderation when it comes to alcohol. "There's no evidence, unless you are driving, that drinking alcohol in limited quantities is bad for you," says Judith S. Stern, Sc.D., a registered dietitian and professor of nutrition at the University of California, Davis. Alcohol in excess (more than two drinks per day) is another story: It will destroy livers as well as lives.

PRACTICE SAFE EATING

While many people are worried about pesticides on fruit and vegetables, the experts rated it 34 out of 44 on their list of priorities.

More than three-quarters of the nutritionists thought it wise to avoid raw foods, particularly eggs, meat and seafood. Raw eggs and chicken can harbor salmonella bacteria, a common cause of food poisoning. Raw seafood can harbor viruses or parasites. Buy only from a reputable dealer, or avoid raw seafood altogether.

GET MORE FIBER

Insoluble or soluble? It doesn't matter how you get your fiber. What's important is that you do get it. "People eat so little fiber, we'll take anything," says Dr. Blackburn. "Whatever you can find—some peas in your stew—put them in!"

A high-fiber diet fills you up without filling you out, keeps you regular, helps lower your cholesterol level and may help reduce the risk of colon cancer. The nutritionists advocate getting at least 20 grams per day. A breakfast of oatmeal, whole-wheat toast, a pear and a banana would give you more than half that amount. The highest-fiber foods are fruits, vegetables, whole grains and legumes.

MORE SURF, LESS TURF

Fish is lower in saturated fat than meat, and the oil in fish—especially cold-water varieties such as salmon and mackerel—helps your cardiovascular system by keeping blood from clotting and preventing hardening of the arteries. If you do eat meat, the experts recommend limiting portions to three or four ounces, choosing lean cuts such as flank steak and using low-fat cooking methods such as broiling and braising.

AVOID FADS

Many nutrition hazards you read or hear about on the 11 o'clock news aren't worth paying attention to, according to our experts. For example, avoiding trans-fatty acids (found in stick margarine) and tropical oils drew only moderate priority ratings from the nutrition authorities, despite their getting big play in the news. Again, it's much more important to lower *total* fat intake.

The experts also said most of us need not worry about sugar. It's a problem for people who are obese (it's got lots of calories but little nutrition) or diabetic (they can't metabolize it properly). For the rest of us, though, avoiding sugar is of only moderate importance.

Rated lowest of all was avoiding irradiated foods—68 percent of respondents put this among the Probably Worthless, right down there with avoiding charred or blackened foods. Neither appear to pose any significant health risk.

• •

FOOD FACTS, FOOD FADS

Men's Health went to over 300 experts and asked them what makes for a healthy diet. Here are the actions they recommend. The higher the number, the greater its importance.

Score	Action
High Priority	
79	Control calories to control weight
76	Reduce all dietary fats
71	Increase physical activity
71	Enjoy your food
70	Eat a balanced diet
69	Get the RDAs of vitamins and minerals
65	Reduce saturated fats
65	Limit alcohol intake
63	Avoid raw eggs, meat and seafood
62	Boost fiber to 20 grams per day
61	Eat fish instead of meat
Low Priority	
16	Make breakfast the biggest meal of the day
14	Avoid irradiated foods
13	Avoid charred or blackened foods

• •

STOP WATCHING THE CLOCK

Our experts gave only a moderate priority rating to avoiding snacks and eating three square meals a day. It seems the nutrition masters are trying to tell us something: What you eat is much more important than how or when you eat.

—*Susan Zarrow*

Stack the Deck

Want to know how to build a better sandwich?
Here are some healthy hand-held meals
for the well-breaded lifestyle.

• •

FROM ITS VERY BEGINNING, the sandwich has been the ultimate in regular-guy food. John Montagu, the Fourth Earl of Sandwich, invented this prototypical nosh not out of culinary genius but because he was a lunatic card player. Deep into a 24-hour game and reluctant to leave the table for sustenance, he instructed a servant to bring him a slab of beef between pieces of toast, and the sandwich was born. More than three centuries later, this hand-held meal remains the salvation of men reluctant to leave the card table, the sports arena or the chair in front of the TV.

Unfortunately, many of today's sandwiches are not much more healthful than old Montagu's. Usually we eat whatever will fit between two slices of bread, from fat- and sodium-laden cured lunch meats to artery-clogging mayonnaise.

We'd never suggest that you abandon sandwiches altogether. It wouldn't do much good if we did. Americans love sandwiches. In fact, a survey found that sandwiches account for half of all lunches eaten in restaurants, 30 percent of all dinners and 19 percent of all *breakfasts*. Instead of admonishing you to quit sandwiches, we'd like to offer some advice on how to build them better.

FROM THE BOTTOM UP

A good place to begin is with the foundation of the sandwich: the bread. Even the spongiest, whitest of white breads supplies healthful complex carbohydrates, but it's best to go with whole-grain varieties, which offer the additional benefit of two times the fiber of plain white bread. For our money, whole-grain bread also tastes better.

You can get whole-grain breads in fat, crusty loaves from bakeries, and you can also get them in neat, sliced and packaged versions at your grocer's. Both are fine, but if you prefer the latter type, check out the ingredient list and buy only those breads that have a whole grain at the top of the label. On the other hand, don't let your imagination stop at bread that comes in loaves. You can also buy whole-grain bagels, rolls, English muffins and pita bread.

Now that we've got the foundation of our sandwich, it's time to select the filling. Fish and seafood are the healthiest choices, since most of them tend to be lower in fat than meat. A simple broiled fish fillet makes a great sandwich filler. Three ounces of cod contains only 89 calories and less than a gram of fat. Drizzle a little lemon juice on the fillet, pack it between two slices of whole-grain bread, add lettuce and tomato, then paint on a layer of spicy mustard for a delicious, light meal.

CAN THE FAT

If you prefer the convenience of canned seafood, be sure you get water-packed tuna, salmon or sardines rather than the oil-packed versions. The savings in fat are considerable:

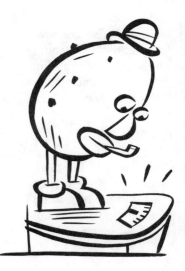

Put Your Spuds on a Diet

It's not the spuds, it's the extras we shovel on that are fattening. Potatoes are low in fat and high in potassium, vitamin C and fiber. Here are some healthy ways to dress them up.

Instead of sour cream, top with plain low-fat yogurt, salsa or a mixture of lemon juice and ground black pepper.

Mash potatoes with buttermilk, which, despite its name, is far lower in fat than whole milk.

If you crave fries, choose thick steak fries. They absorb less oil.

Leave the skin on scalloped potatoes (to keep the fiber high), and use skim milk and just a dab of margarine.

Three ounces of oil-packed chunk tuna usually contains 18 grams of fat, about 16½ grams more than the water-packed kind.

For low-fat sandwich fillings, things that swim are followed closely by things with wings, specifically chicken and turkey. A three-ounce portion of skinless chicken breast— about three slices—weighs in at under four grams of fat, while turkey is the champion with just over two grams.

Some sliced deli meats are okay, but most are loaded with fat. Stay away from standard cured lunch meats like bologna, salami and hard sausage or any others that we used to call "mystery meats" when we were kids. They generally deliver about 20 to 25 grams of fat per three- to four-slice portion. (To keep within the suggested health guidelines of the American Heart Association, a man of average weight and appetite should consume no more than 80 grams of fat in an entire day.) It does little good to switch to the "lite" versions of bologna made from turkey or chicken. Even though they're cleverly described on the packages as being one-third lower in fat than the original, they still weigh in at 15 to 20 grams per three-slice serving, which means that as much as 80 percent of their calories are from fat. A better bet at the deli department is to choose meats like boiled ham, roast turkey or lean roast beef, all of which are relatively low in fat.

If you favor deli food, it's nearly impossible to avoid the food additives known as nitrates. These are added to prevent spoilage and retain the appetizing color of the meat. The whole issue of whether or not nitrates are a major risk factor for some types of cancer is unanswered as yet. Still, the American Cancer Society recommends limiting your intake of nitrate-cured meats, unless they have vitamin C compounds added. Researchers think that the vitamin C may keep nitrates from turning into cancer-causing chemicals. Vitamin C has been added if the label includes mention of *ascorbic acid, sodium ascorbate* or *sodium erythrobate.*

Most people don't consider a sandwich a sandwich without some cheese thrown in. That might seem like a problem, since about 50 to 70 percent of the calories from many cheeses are from fat. One solution is simply to use less. Will two or three slices make the sandwich taste that much better than a single slice will? For us, the answer is no. Cheese is very flavorful, and a little goes a long way.

It's also a good idea to use lower-fat cheeses whenever possible. A slice of Cheddar will contribute about ten grams of fat to your sandwich, but mozzarella adds only six grams. Even better, try a *part-skim* version of mozzarella, which cuts down the fat content by about another 20 percent. Similar savings can be found with low-fat Cheddar, Monterey Jack or Swiss. At these levels, the amount of fat you are adding is small enough to justify the flavor benefits of cheese. Cheese also supplies significant amounts of protein and calcium to your meal.

ADMIRABLE ADDITIONS

Next we come to the two areas in which imagination serves up the greatest rewards for sandwich eaters: vegetables and condiments. Both of these ingredients have traditionally been used to fill the important role of moistening the other filling ingredients, but they can also do much more.

Tomatoes and lettuce are fine sandwich garnishes, but it pays to extend your repertoire. Try slightly bitter greens such as arugula or watercress, which add more taste complexity than iceberg lettuce (and more nutrients, too). Add vegetables such as shredded cabbage, alfalfa sprouts or strips of bell pepper, which give a nice crunchy texture as well as good flavor. To give the basic roast beef sandwich a lift, throw on some watercress, which contributes a little flavor, a little crunch and a little moisture.

Now we come to condiments. Here the dictates of flavor and healthfulness combine, for the one condiment that you should permanently leave out of your sandwiches is bland and cholesterol-laden mayonnaise. ("As a general rule, healthy sandwiches should crunch, not ooze," says *Men's Health* nutritionist Anita Hirsch.) Instead of mayonnaise, with 11 grams of fat per tablespoon, use one of the new low-fat or nonfat mayonnaise-type dressings or stronger-flavored Dijon mustard, horseradish, bottled chutney or cranberry sauce. Just by way of comparison, you would have to eat 30 cups of cranberry sauce to equal the amount of fat in one tablespoon of mayonnaise. Horseradish, the condiment of choice for a roast beef sandwich, has no measurable fat at all, so you save the entire

• •

FILLING STATION

You don't have to count calories or grams of fat if all your sand-wich ingredients are lean. Mix and match these fixings for an easy low-fat meal by picking one item from each of the four cate-gories below. Add as many extras as you like.

BREAD

- Bagel
- English muffin
- Flour tortilla
- French bread
- Italian roll
- Kaiser roll
- Pita bread
- Whole-grain bread

CONDIMENTS

- Fruit butters
- Flavored vinegars
- Herbal soft cheese
- Horseradish
- Low-fat salad dressing
- Mustard
- Reduced-calorie mayonnaise
- Red beets, grated
- Tahini dressing

FILLINGS

- Chicken salad
- Grilled chicken cutlet
- Low-fat sliced cheese
- Nonbreaded fish fillet
- Seafood salad
- Sliced lean meat
- Smoked salmon
- Tuna salad

EXTRAS

- Carrot, grated
- Cucumber slices
- Lettuce
- Low-fat cheese, grated
- Mushrooms, sliced
- Onion
- Red and green cabbage, grated
- Sesame seeds, toasted
- Spinach
- Sprouts
- Sweet pepper rings
- Tomato slices
- Watercress

• •

11 grams of fat you would have eaten with that tablespoon of mayonnaise.

So there you have it, in honor of the earl, a full-fledged roast beef sandwich—three slices of lean roast beef, a slice of low-fat Swiss cheese, lettuce, tomato and horseradish on whole-wheat bread—that weighs in at 424 calories and less than 14 grams of fat. It's a hearty meal that won't make you feel like a nitpicking calorie-counter.

If you start feeling a bit frisky and want to experiment with some ethnic cuisines, try one of these sandwiches.

Italian. For an update on the submarine sandwich, paint a crusty roll with a bit of whole-grain mustard and top it with three ounces of chicken breast, a couple of thin-sliced artichoke hearts and a few cured black olives or sun-dried tomatoes.

Mexican. Mix a can of water-packed tuna with the juice of half a lime, a tablespoon of chopped fresh cilantro and a teaspoon of chili powder or your favorite Caribbean hot sauce. Wrap it all up in a tortilla.

Greek. Into a whole-wheat pita, put two slices of grilled eggplant. Add diced red bell peppers, garlic and watercress or lettuce. Sprinkle with lemon juice.

—John Willoughby

Get Your Cholesterol Down—Or Else!

You're sort of slim, sort of fit, and the doctor has told you it's now or never. Here's what you can do when your cholesterol test comes back high.

• •

MY FACE MUST HAVE gone ashen that day six months ago at my health club when Lou read me my results at the while-u-wait cholesterol screening. Lou is the club's equipment manager. Four times a year he turns into a sweat-suited cardiologist when he runs the portable testing machine the club sponsors. He had just told me my number was 233.

"Hey, don't get so bent out of shape," he said cheerily.
"It's not like you're gonna die."

Wrong, barbell head, I thought, a lump of worry caged inside my ribs. I *am* gonna die. The only mystery is when. It had been a less than stellar day to begin with. I'd cut my gums flossing too vigorously, driven off from the self-serve pump with my gas cap on the roof and found my secretary circulating a caricature of me as a balding infant in fully loaded diapers. In fact, it was only because I needed the satisfaction of getting one thing right that I'd let them stick me with that needle at the health club.

After all, I had reasoned, at 35, I'm still in the pink of health: trim (6 feet, 160 nonsmoking pounds), fit (I run four miles three times a week and play squash once or twice) and reasonably diet-conscious (almost no red meat, 2 percent milk on my banana and shredded wheat, light lunches so I can keep from drooling over my work in the afternoon). I hadn't had my cholesterol tested since my last physical, two years ago. All I remembered was that my doctor had said it was okay.

Yet now, even as I watched the back of Lou's crew-cut head while he loaded my slide into a machine resembling a bowling-ball polisher, my own sweaty palms dismantled my confidence. I was thinking that all the men on both sides of my family had died of heart trouble. The machine hummed while its red digital readout flashed past 100, 150, then 200. This was like the Wheel of Fortune in hell—and there was no Vanna anywhere in sight.

Anything below 200, I'd been told, was basically cool. From 200 to 240 was borderline dangerous, a car with bald tires and bad brakes. Anything above 240 was grizzly country, a highwire act with no net. Finally the digital devil froze at 233—somewhere in the high foothills of the Coronary Range—and I did, too. It was, I think, at that moment that I crossed over from the "young" column into the one marked "middle age." My body, not unlike a girlfriend with whom one lives comfortably and unconsciously for years, was suddenly packed and standing at the door. Better be nice to me, it was saying, or I'm out of here.

BANISH THE BADDIES

That night I threw out the Häagen-Dazs Swiss Almond Vanilla and the frozen pepperoni French-bread pizzas lurking at the back of the freezer. I bought oatmeal, skim milk and half a grocery cart of fruits and vegetables. If a hair shirt would have helped, I would've gotten one of those, too. I also called my doctor, who told me those while-u-wait cholesterol tests are not particularly reliable, not least of all because a true reading of your LDL cholesterol (the so-called bad kind) requires you to fast the night before.

Two days later, after a test at the doctor's office, my heart had a new number: 224, lower than the health-club reading but still on the high side. "Look," my internist told me, "it's not a good number; it should be lower, but it's nothing to get flipped out about. If you were fat and sedentary, things might be different. I might consider putting you on a cholesterol-lowering drug. But you're not. The important thing for you to do is work on your diet, cut down on the animal fats and tropical oils. Then we'll check your cholesterol level again in three months and see where we stand."

The doctor also gave me the name of a nutritionist I could talk with if I wanted more information. I did.

Susan Natale, a registered dietitian, teaches cardiac nutrition classes at the Washington Hospital Center. Most of her patients have had their hearts stop beating at one time or other, an experience that tends to convince them of the need to change their diets. She has the directness one finds in hospital personnel everywhere.

"You've got three things going against you that you can't do much about," she told me over the phone. "One, you're male. And men have a greater incidence of heart disease than women. Two, you're getting older. The older you get, the more likely you are to have heart trouble. And three, your family history, from what I gather, is bad. Lotsa heart attacks. That's the bad news."

GOOD NEWS AND BAD NEWS

The good news was that there were two other risk factors I *could* do something about—exercise and diet. I exercise regularly, which she told me was a plus. In fact, the Centers for Disease Control say that sedentary living, not high cholesterol, is the leading preventable cause of coronary death in this country—sedentary people have twice as many heart attacks as those who get even mild regular exercise. As for my diet, she said it sounded pretty good, but could be better. Furthermore, my blood pressure was low—another good sign.

Sue is a busy woman, but I kept her on the phone for about half an hour talking mainly about nutrition. We discussed LDL (bad) cholesterol and HDL (good) cholesterol (see "Good vs. Bad Cholesterol" on page 48). She essentially reinforced what my doctor had told me: Avoid animal fats and anything high in saturated fats, such as palm, palm kernel and coconut oils. Eat lots of fruits, vegetables and whole grains.

Okay, I thought, lose 24 points and you're in the clear. Willpower time.

Although I'd long since weaned myself of the daily meat habit and had found it fairly easy to cut back in general on high-cholesterol foods, eliminating them altogether was going to be difficult. Like most American children, I was raised hooked up to a cow. Cookies and milk were a tradition dating back to nursery school. And when that Good Humor truck bell rang outside on summer nights, a whole brain lobe went ballistic. Chocolate malts had an equally long lineage.

I knew I couldn't kick dairy products cold turkey. At first I tried skim milk over my cereal and banana, but it was so sad that I stopped. The problem with skim is you can see through it and your eye forewarns your stomach that what is coming is not really milk but dairy plasma. Even 1 percent is opaque by comparison, so I compromised and used it.

Sugar, the nutritional plutonium of the 1970s, is making a comeback these days. They may be empty calories, but they are fat-free, sweet ones. I decided I would go for it when the craving for bad food got too strong. The key would be finding sweet, satisfying foods that weren't overladen with fat.

LEARNING TO READ LABELS

I became a food-label reader. I cased out the candy machine at my office and said a fond farewell to fat-laden

• •

GOOD VS. BAD CHOLESTEROL

Pure cholesterol is an odorless, white, waxy, powdery substance. You can't taste it in the foods you eat, and you can't see it. Despite all its bad press, your body needs it to make essential body substances such as cell walls and hormones.

Like other fats, cholesterol won't mix with water. Therefore, to carry cholesterol and fat in the blood, the body "wraps" them in protein packages. This compound is called a lipoprotein.

Low-density lipoproteins (LDLs) contain the greatest amounts of cholesterol. They're believed to be responsible for depositing cholesterol on artery walls.

High-density lipoproteins (HDLs) contain the greatest amounts of protein and the least amounts of cholesterol. They're believed to remove cholesterol from artery walls and carry it away to the liver for reprocessing and removal from the body. To better understand any total cholesterol reading, it's useful to know what portion is HDL and what portion is LDL (see the table below).

Higher levels of the HDL—the good stuff—are usually found in people who exercise regularly, don't smoke and stay at a desirable weight.

LDL		**HDL**	
Level	**Risk**	**Level**	**Risk**
160 or over	High	under 35	Additional risk
130-159	Borderline-high	35 or over	Desirable
under 130	Desirable		

Total Cholesterol	
Level	**Risk**
240 or over	High
200-239	Borderline-high
under 200	Desirable

• •

Reese's Peanut Butter Cups, my former favorite. I welcomed Cracker Jacks ("sugar, corn syrup, popcorn, molasses, salt and soya lecithin," only 120 calories per box, 22 grams of carbohydrate, 3 grams fat). Hard pretzels contain only 10 percent fat, and they too joined my list of safe bets. Oreos, which you might think are harmless, actually contain lard, among other ingredients. I placed them on restricted status.

As for the holy trinity of fruits, whole grains and vegetables, it was a struggle at first to be a believer. I thought of them in the same way I thought of G-rated movies, notable primarily for what they leave out: barbecue, bacon, warm Brie with almonds, Slim Jims, eggs Benedict, Personal Pan Supreme pizza.

I could go on.

As I would load up my lunch tray at the Healthy Hut salad bar with rice, steamed broccoli and cantaloupe—Billy's Pit Beef was now strictly off-limits—I tried to tell myself it wasn't so bad. Outside I was smiling; inside I was crying. It wasn't so much that I missed the ribs. I missed what used to come after the ribs—rich, lovely desserts. I mourned the death of pastry of all kinds, including the German and Italian but most dearly the French.

GUILTY BUT HAPPY

Once every two weeks or so, alone with my sin, I would yield. There is a bakery near where I work that makes a napoleon that Napoleon himself would have esteemed. The crème oozes out under a hundred stories of sheaf pastry collapsing beneath my teeth like a high-rise in an earthquake movie. I made it a point to take my pleasure crudely, standing on the sidewalk in full view of strangers, savaging what I should be savoring. It was heavenly. Afterward I felt guilty. And happy.

Mostly, I was good. Certainly more good than not. I haven't been in a McDonald's in months. When I was drawn toward the office candy machine, I didn't even look at the high-fat choices. I got a box of Cracker Jacks or dumped a prepackaged lowfat hot chocolate into my coffee, trying to push the chocolate and caffeine buttons while hopping nimbly over the fat.

It became easier with time. I struggled with the feeling that I was being unfairly deprived. Then, at a certain point, I made my peace with it. The cravings for fatty foods, for pastries, for chocolate ice cream began to dissipate. In fact, after about six weeks of eating light, going for that napoleon wasn't as pleasurable as I'd anticipated. I imagined it congealing in a big lump in my stomach. I also noticed my overall energy level was improving from lighter fare. A lunch of barbecued ribs, french fries and creamy potato salad at Billy's used to leave me ready for a two-hour nap—and next to useless in that afternoon meeting.

THE HEART OF THE MATTER

So mostly I stick to good food. My chief motivation for improving my diet is the new awareness I have of my heart itself. It feels more exposed now, unprotected, a fragile dove beating its wings in my rib cage. My idea of a good workout once centered on the muscles I wanted other people to see: my sculpted deltoids, my bulging arms, my tapered legs. All of a sudden that is losing its allure. Now I am oriented toward the one muscle I hope never to see, which has become the most real of them all. I run it harder than ever when I work out, hoping to scour the arterial walls of plaque. I remind myself that there are guys older than I who can run a marathon in two hours and 20 minutes; twenty-six 5½-minute miles clicked off back-to-back. After I take my heart out for a run, I want to stroke its forehead as you would a good horse's and whisper encouragement to it. Good run, big fella, good going, very smooth.

Because I was anxious, I got retested two weeks shy of the three-month wait my doctor recommended. My new number was 194, a significant improvement. I was coming out of the Coronary Mountains, back down to the foothills. Some would say I was already there. But a little knowledge can be a strong motivator. Given my heredity, the thing that's going to finally do me in is my heart. The way I figure it, the lower my number, the longer I get to hang around.

In two more months, I punched in at 176. I wish they gave out little patches I could sew on my gym shorts to identify me as a member of the Clean Artery Club. I'm aiming for 150, but in my mind I'm out of the danger zone. This, in a way, makes

HOW TO TEST YOUR CHOLESTEROL

Depending on how, where and when you get your cholesterol tested, the reading can vary by as much as 40 points in either direction. To get the most reliable reading, follow these guidelines.

Don't do it at the mall. Those quickie finger-stick tests can be wildly inaccurate for a number of reasons, ranging from poor or miscalibrated testing equipment to contamination of the blood sample. Instead have blood drawn through a needle at a lab certified by the Centers for Disease Control.

Get repeat tests. Even if you go to the best labs, readings can still vary because of changes in your body's cholesterol level from day to day or even from hour to hour. "Although these variations are usually under 10 percent, if your first reading is extremely high or is borderline, it pays to get tested two or three times—a couple of days apart—and take an average," says Basil Rifkind, M.D., chief of the Lipid Metabolism and Atherogenesis Branch at the National Heart, Lung and Blood Institute in Washington, D.C.

Don't sweat it. Get your cholesterol checked before you exercise. You lose water when you exert yourself vigorously, and as a result your blood becomes more concentrated. That can lead to higher cholesterol readings.

Stick to your regular diet. Although one or two high-fat meals may not have much effect on your blood cholesterol levels, a consistent pattern of such eating can boost your numbers. Similarly, if you've been following an unusually low-fat diet recently, your numbers may be unrealistically low.

Sit down, but not for long. Have a seat before having blood drawn, but not for more than 5 minutes. Cholesterol readings decline by as much as 10 to 15 percent in people who've been resting longer than 20 minutes.

If you're laid up, don't do it. Any surgery or illness—even a cold or the flu—can alter the composition of your blood and throw your cholesterol reading out of whack. The Laboratory Standardization Panel of the National Cholesterol Education Program advises waiting two months after illness or surgery before being tested.

things harder. Will I be able to stick with the program? I stoke my self-control with pop-psychology tricks: visualizing the glistening white plaque deposits from a blood-red steamship round of beef, seeing *pâté de canard* as a ribbon of sludge encircling my struggling heart. Some of it's just plain discipline. On a restaurant menu, I have trained myself to ignore the meat and head for the fish or salads. I ask for the dill butter sauce on the side with my salmon, and I eat the rolls without butter. At a cookout, if everyone else is having a hamburger, I will, too. (I don't want to come off like a jerk.) But I'll just have one, and I'll make a mental note that I have used up my animal-fat allotment for the next day or two.

The strongest motivator is the knowledge that, unless I suffer a fatal slip on a cake of soap or accidentally get mowed down in a drive-by shooting, the condition of my heart is likely to be the dominant factor in how long I to get to hang around before I move on to that big pastry shop in the sky. When you put it in those terms, it's not all that hard to have oatmeal for breakfast instead of eggs.

—Bill Heavey

It's the Better Thing to Do

Oat bran may get all the press coverage, but psyllium is the superstar when it comes to lowering your cholesterol.

● ●

GET ME HOLLYWOOD. Time for *Mary Poppins II*. We get Julie Andrews. She sings. But forget that spoonful of sugar stuff. Times change. This time it's: "A spoonful of psyllium helps the cholesterol go down…" Think of the commercial tie-ins. Memo to Madison Avenue: We'll blow Wilford Brimley right off the tube…

Okay, so we're making lowering cholesterol sound suspiciously easy. But we figure anything worth doing is worth doing the easy way, and besides, this psyllium stuff really seems to work.

Oat bran and psyllium are both sources of soluble fiber, which helps lower cholesterol. Lately, studies have questioned whether oat bran's effect comes from the fiber itself, or from the fact that an oat-bran muffin simply fills you up, making you less likely to tackle an Egg McMuffin afterward. Either way, psyllium is a much better source of soluble fiber than oat bran.

Psyllium is a grain that is grown in India and the Mediterranean, and it happens to be nature's all-time greatest source of soluble fiber. It takes about eight teaspoons of oat bran (or about 1½ bowls of oatmeal) to match the amount of soluble fiber in a single teaspoon of psyllium. Of course, if you're a label reader, none of this is news to you; psyllium is used in bulk-forming laxatives (such as Metamucil and Fiberall), and recently it's been added to some breakfast cereals.

JUST WHAT THE DOCTOR ORDERED

All of which seem to be just what the doctors are ordering. "We encourage people to use psyllium in addition to changing their diet," says Donald Smith, M.D., a lipids and metabolism researcher at the Mount Sinai Medical Center in New York. "Soluble fiber really does reduce the harmful form

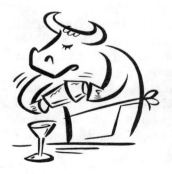

High-Calcium Cocktails

You can reduce high blood pressure by eating more low-fat dairy products and drinking lots of fortified orange juice, suggest studies out of Arizona State University. Men who ate a high-calcium diet (600 milligrams more than the Recommended Dietary Allowance) for six weeks saw their high blood pressure readings drop dramatically.

of cholesterol, whether you get the fiber from fruits, vegetables, beans, grains or psyllium."

In one study, men who ate a typical American diet took a teaspoon of psyllium three times a day for eight weeks and dropped their levels of harmful cholesterol by 20 percent. (Every 1 percent decrease in cholesterol means a 2 percent decrease in the incidence of heart attacks.) In another study, harmful cholesterol decreased an additional 8 percent among men who ate a low-fat diet plus psyllium, as compared to those who just dieted.

Psyllium may also help you lose weight, according to George Blackburn, M.D., Ph.D., chief of the Nutrition/Metabolism Laboratory at New England Deaconess Hospital in Boston. High-fiber foods take longer to digest, so your stomach feels full longer and you eat less.

Just don't take that as license to eat anything you want as long as you follow it with a few teaspoons of fiber. "There's a rumor going around that you can lose weight on ice cream and candy bars as long as you send them down the hatch with some fiber," says Dr. Blackburn. "The claim is that the fiber will escort a large portion of the calories out the back door. That's a wild exaggeration."

When you're ready to lower your cholesterol, the first step is to switch to a low-fat diet and to include some oat bran in your meals. Then, says Peter Kwiterovich, Jr., M.D., author of *Beyond Cholesterol: The Johns Hopkins Complete Guide for Avoiding Heart Disease,* if your cholesterol level is still borderline high (200 to 240) or high (over 240) ask your doctor if you should be taking one teaspoon of powdered psyllium three times a day to achieve an additional reduction. Metamucil is probably the best-known psyllium product, but there are dozens of brands of psyllium in powdered and tablet form at pharmacies and health-food stores. Dr. Smith of Mount Sinai recommends stirring powdered psyllium into an eight-ounce glass of water before meals.

If you begin your day with a high-fiber breakfast (a one-ounce serving of Kellogg's Heartwise cereal, which contains psyllium, gives you close to a teaspoon of soluble fiber), you can skip your morning teaspoon of psyllium and take only two teaspoons later.

EASY DOES IT

Just don't overdo it, warns Dr. Blackburn. More fiber is not necessarily better, and too much can cause stomach upset, gas and diarrhea.

And what if you have no reason to assume you're among the unlucky one in five American men with a cholesterol level in the risky zones above 200?

"I'd recommend taking psyllium anyway," says Larry Bell, M.D., of the University of Minnesota, whose psyllium research appeared in the *Journal of the American Medical Association.* "Whether it lowers your cholesterol or not, many health groups recommend that we get more fiber in our diets."

Remember, the longer your cholesterol stays elevated, the greater your danger of heart disease. A diet that's low in fat and high in soluble fiber, including psyllium, is a way to eat smart and protect your heart.

—*Douglas Carpenter*

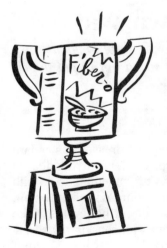

Fiber Champs

These ten foods are loaded with fiber.

1. All Bran with Extra Fiber, ½ cup: 13.8 grams
2. Kidney beans, cooked, ½ cup: 6.9 grams
3. Wheat "lite" bread, 2 slices: 5.6 grams
4. Turnips, cooked, ½ cup: 4.8 grams
5. Green peas, frozen, cooked, ½ cup: 4.3 grams
6. Pears, canned, ½ cup: 3.7 grams
7. Raspberries, fresh, 1 cup: 3.3 grams
8. French-style green beans, cooked, ½ cup: 2.8 grams
9. Granny Smith apple, 1 small: 2.8 grams
10. Popcorn, 3 cups: 2.0 grams

Part 3

MEN AT EASE

Go Your Own Way

Is it time for separate vacations? Family vacations are well and good, but sometimes a man's got to get away alone.

••••••••••••••••••••

MY WIFE, OUR TWO CHILDREN and I, all dressed in standard issue tourist clothing, are at Epcot Center, surrounded by cheerful and informative displays having something to do with The Wonderful World of Communication. As a family unit, however, we are communicating about on the level of Koko the talking ape. I've had it up to here with chasing my seven-year-old son all over the fake-futuristic landscape. My four-year-old daughter is indignant because I will not buy her the guy who walks around dressed up as Goofy, or anything else she happens to lay eyes upon. And my wife, who has meticulously planned the trip using Stephen Birnbaum's guidebook—which lays out the complete strategy for mastering Disney World, including the correct times of day to stand in line at various unforgettable attractions—does not feel I have taken her efforts seriously enough.

So there the two of us stand, our noses six inches apart, fighting in the AT&T Pavilion, while the kids run off to God knows where. I'm arguing that we should all just get loose and wander around. She is arguing that you can't do Disney World that way. You've got to have goals, a timetable, a whole strategic plan. You need drive, focus, willpower. This is not a vacation, she seems to be saying; it's a job.

By 8 o'clock at night, we're both exhausted. We have to catch the picturesque monorail back to the picturesque hotel, but it's a long walk to the station, and neither one of us is exactly sure where it is. I've been lugging around a cutely decorated bag full of—I don't know, Mickey's Whoopie Cushions—for hours, and I just want to go to bed. But we've got work to do, more happiness to achieve, great vistas of pleasure to stand in line for. We've got to make sure we get our money's worth for our all-day passes.

I can hardly wait.

Now, I'm not suggesting that a father should not sometimes allow himself to be walked upon (metaphorically speaking) in order to acquaint his children with the world's pleasures. I'm not suggesting that a family vacation at Disney World (or Six Flags Over Texas, or Dollywood, or Sea World, or Carburetor World, or wherever) is a complete waste of money. What I am suggesting is that, if this is the only sort of vacation you ever allow yourself, you will probably wind up committing suicide before you normally would have.

RECHARGE YOUR BATTERIES

Which brings me to my point: Every now and then, when you go on vacation, you need to leave the lady and the kids behind. You must not allow yourself to feel guilty about this, either. This is not abandonment, this is renewal. When you come back, I guarantee you'll be the better for it, or your money back. Everybody else in your life will be the better for it, too, because they probably need to get away from you as desperately as you need to get away from them.

Several months after our family outing to Florida, I took my own good advice. My buddy Jim and I sailed out to an uninhabited barrier island off the coast of North Carolina and spent four days camping in the dunes, fishing, lolling, philosophizing and generally working hard to accomplish absolutely nothing. We got greasy and tired and sunburned and windburned. We survived a series of sea squalls that collapsed my tent in the night, caught ghost crabs and bluefish and sharks, bodysurfed in the moonlight, figured out the rhythm of the wind and the tides and sunrise and moonrise, and several times got to laughing so hard we may have come perilously close to death itself.

This trip was the fourth in a dramatic series starring Jim and me. It's sort of a pact we've made, involving the two of us and water. Every summer for the past four years, we've gone to find some interesting body of water and get seriously involved in it for a couple of days. One summer we canoed a stretch of flat water on the weird, mystical, north-flowing New River in southern Virginia. Another time we did the northern reaches of the Susquehanna in upstate New York. And yet another time we camped and canoed among the forested river islands of the James in central Virginia, taking my boy along to celebrate his seventh birthday.

CHEAP FUN

One thing all these trips had in common (besides water) is that they didn't cost much. The last time out, we spent all of $250 (gas, food, bait, rum) in four days, setting us each back around $30 a day. We squeezed a phenomenal amount of pleasure out of every penny. When we got back home, I was left with a feeling of physical exhaustion and spiritual rehabilitation that was better than a visit to Lourdes.

The experience of that trip was summed up and symbolized by a hat. I'd felt in serious need of a good hat for this trip, the sort of hat you couldn't buy but could only be given. On the drive down, Jim obliged by handing me a truly excellent bit of headgear he'd gotten off a roadie in George Thorogood's R&B band. It was one of those adjustable ball caps, all black except for the white outline of an electric guitar and the word *Destroyers*. Except to sleep and swim, I don't think I took that hat off once in four days. It came to represent a new, changed self, a vacation self. Wearing it gave me the feeling that I'd actually gone somewhere. When I got home, I took the hat off and hung it on a chair. It'll stay there until that old vacation self comes back.

The thing is this: When you take your whole family along, it makes it all the more difficult to open yourself up to the unexpected, to take risks, to hang one over the edge. A typical family vacation is usually just a matter of transporting all your old habits and attitudes (plus half your possessions) to a new location, generating huge credit-card bills and then going home. In order to escape a daily routine that's overscheduled, stressed-out and fraught with goals and deadlines, for instance, we'll go someplace like Disney World, which requires a 150-page guidebook. We emerge fundamentally unchanged from this experience, except for being more tired than ever—and poorer. The real agenda behind these vacations, in fact, is not about being changed at all but about avoiding change.

THE THRILL OF THE UNEXPECTED

For Jim and me, though, the whole point was *not* to know exactly what was coming next. We didn't dread the unexpected; we welcomed it. We worked it right into the agenda, by sketching out a basic scheme (head down to Cape Lookout with tents, fishing gear and a boat) but making sure to keep all the details as vague as possible. That way, something surprising was bound to happen. The Plan was so broadly—might I say brilliantly—conceived that anything that happened was a part of it. No matter what came next, The Plan was running like a fine watch, and everything was right on schedule. When The Plan went plunging wildly off the tracks, well, that's exactly what we hoped would happen.

In this case, the unexpected took the form of weather. For about a week before we left Virginia, the weather reports from the Carolina coast were a trifle on the damp side: A huge low-pressure system was stalled in the area, producing heavy rain, localized squalls and thundershowers. The morning before we were supposed to leave, we decided to postpone the trip. It was only prudent, we figured. It took us about three hours to recognize the utter foolishness of prudence. Life is short and uncertain, and if we didn't go now, we might never go. We'd both be 65 before we knew it. Besides, we just felt like it.

It was warm and sunny when we left home, but by the time we reached the coast, it was apparent that every once in a while the weatherman gets it right. We were driving directly into a vast and majestic electrical storm. Immense panoramas of evil darkness, roiling with menace. Then, quite mysteriously, we drove right out of it. By the time we reached the water, it was no longer raining.

We off-loaded the boat and settled her in the water. The vessel was a 12-foot flat-bottomed dory that Jim and his brother

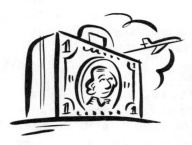

The Thrifty Traveler

Here are some money-saving tips for life on the road.

■ If you order from hotel room service and add a tip, you may be overcharging yourself. Many hotels already include a 15 percent gratuity on room-service bills.

■ If you're quoted a hotel room rate two weeks before your trip, call back *one* week before your trip and check to see if the rate has changed. You may save as much as $50 a night. Many hotels are adopting an airline-like system of adjusting rates according to availability.

■ A group may be smaller than you think when it comes to airlines. Group rates are available for as few as ten passengers on many airlines. The group rate could save you $70 per ticket.

■ The airline allows you only two pieces of luggage without extra charges, but what if you have four cases? Go to the airport's curbside drop-off and leave two cases there. Then go pick up your tickets and check your other two cases there.

had built by hand in Oregon. She had a sail that could be unfurled in the event of wind, but everything was dead calm now, eerily calm, and it looked as if we'd have to row the four miles across the sound to Cape Lookout.

"You gon' drown, boys!" an old guy bawled, sitting in a nearby pickup wasting his life. "It's gon' squall, ain't you heard?" We pushed off anyway, hoping the storm would hold its breath till we got across.

YOU KNOW WHEN YOUR HEART HAS ARRIVED

The real goal of a vacation is to get that feeling of actually having been somewhere, of having temporarily taken leave of your everyday life. But that sensation is an interior experience, a matter of the heart, and it doesn't necessarily have anything to do with spending lots of money or even physically going someplace. You can spend a week in Cancun but somehow never get away. "Getting away" has more to do with getting away from yourself, or at least from your obligations, and neither of those things has anything to do with geography.

Which is why occasionally taking a vacation free of wife and family is almost automatically magic. You're stripping away all your ordinary, task-specific selves—father, husband, lover, slave of children—as if you were shedding a series of overcoats. You're breaking free of the thousand daily reminders that keep all those selves intact and just walking away from the whole thing. That's when the trip begins.

When you take your family along, though, it's almost like loading your whole house on your back. You're taking the thousand daily reminders right along with you. (A friend of mine rented a villa in Italy and took his entire family there for the summer but came back in a few weeks because the whole experience was just like home, only immeasurably more difficult.)

MEN ALONE

Another selling point for the kind of vacation I'm talking about is that—equal rights be damned—there are times when men need the company of male friends. There's some kind of primitive magic in returning to the circle of your own kind, and there's no need to feel guilty about that, either. Up in Minnesota, the big attraction of ice fishing is basically that guys can go out there and sit in a hut, drink beer and get away from women for a while. The fact that we seem to have lost sight of this shows just how alienated from ourselves we really are.

But, hey, I'm not here to pick a fight. I'm here to get you to go with me.

Core Sound was mostly sandy-bottomed and shallow, dotted with little grassy islands riotous with birds. Jim rowed, I fished. In the still, dark water among the islands, I hooked three little ones with a golden spoon, then released them. Across the water, on Shackleford Banks, wild ponies romped along the beach, filthy and ragged and free. Around us, ominous-looking weather cells swirled and eddied darkly. Occasionally the darkness unleashed rain, then it would slow to a patter and stop. If a squall blew up, we could beach the boat on one of the islands, we figured. But for the hour and a half it took to cross, the storm gave us a break. At twilight, we beached the boat on the lee side of Cape Lookout and made camp back among the pines.

Dragging our gear up out of the boat, I sloshed through the outgoing tide, clear and warm as bathwater. If it didn't rain, we'd get a fire going up above the tide mark. Already my skin was beginning to feel briny and coarse from sun and wind and spray. In the pent-up, citified muscles of my back and shoulders, snaps and buckles and hooks seemed to be coming undone. I took a deep, deep breath, as if I were about to take a long, cool drink of water.

I'd come back to the well.

—*Stefan Bechtel*

The Basics of Booze

Can alcohol be part of a normal, healthy life?
Yes, provided you follow these rules.

••••••••••••••••••••••

EVERYONE KNOWS WHAT WISE pundits barkeeps are. So needless to say, we sat up and blinked when the American Bartenders' Association offered this prediction for the 1990s: "Healthy food, moderation and quality will be deciding factors on where, when and how consumers choose to indulge and celebrate."

Actually, we worry a little that the part about healthy food will mean the demise of the Beer-Nuts and pickled eggs at our favorite tavern, but moderation and quality sound pretty smart to us. If you're going to drink, you might as well drink the good stuff, but whether you quaff Coors or Courvoisier, moderation is a secret of successful imbibing. Another is to know what you're getting into before you let the genie out of the bottle.

Here are some of the best tips we know for healthy drinking. Consider them something along the lines of a package insert for using what's fermented or distilled.

Have a slow hand. Many men end up drunk for the simple reason that they didn't give their first drink enough time to kick in before ordering up a second or third. It takes 20 to 30 minutes for alcohol to do its thing, so wait *at least* that long before having another.

Rotate your days of wine and roses. You really shouldn't drink seven days a week, even if you only have a beer or two. Daily drinkers can unknowingly build up a tolerance to alcohol and may gradually increase intake to realize the feelings they used to experience on smaller doses.

After the buzz, cut. The amount you can drink in an hour without getting smashed varies according to body weight, mood, what you've eaten and other factors. To make it simple, limiting yourself to one drink an hour, the rate at which most people metabolize alcohol, will help prevent you from becoming intoxicated. As researchers note, a "drink" is the equivalent of ½ ounce of pure alcohol, the amount contained in one 12-ounce can of beer, a 1-ounce shot of 80-proof liquor or a 4-ounce glass of most wines.

Count to two. Many alcoholism experts, including Arthur Klatsky, M.D., chief of cardiology at Kaiser Permanente Medical Center in Oakland, California, define moderate drinking as no more than two drinks daily. Some research shows that at three drinks a day, the risk for alcohol-related problems—in particular, higher blood pressure and higher mortality rates—starts to rise.

Avoid the grape escape. Alcohol is not an antidepressant. If you've got the blues, booze will "provoke only momentary relief that keeps you from tackling your problems," says Ethan Gorenstein, Ph.D., assistant professor of clinical psychology at Columbia University. Using alcohol as a cure is the first step toward making drinking a disease.

Don't drink to destress. Rather than relieving stress, drinking can actually increase anxiety. If you're going through a particularly tough time, you should be having two drinks *fewer* per week. Judith Wurtman, Ph.D., a researcher at MIT, recommends drinking little or no alcohol on a day when you know you're going to face a stressful situation.

Stay out of New Hampshire. Those folks up there are a bad influence. Their annual beer consumption—51 gallons per person—is the highest in the United States.

Read tomorrow's weather forecast. The hotter it gets and the more active you are under the sun, the more trouble alcohol can cause. Booze fast-forwards dehydration, says Danny Wheat, an assistant trainer for the Texas Rangers. His team often plays in 100° F-plus conditions in Arlington, Texas. "We stress to players that the night before a day game, they should limit alcohol consumption," he says.

Don't guzzle beer to quench a thirst. You've just worked out or finished a ball game. You've got a powerful thirst, and those kegs are glistening in the sun. Wait. Do one thing at a time. Drink water to replace your sweat loss first. Beer is a lousy thirst-quencher in part because it inhibits the release of a hormone responsible for water retention. The result: frequent urination, leading to fluid *loss* rather than fluid replacement, explains nutritionist and registered dietitian Nancy Clark. Not to mention the fact that you may inadvertently end up loaded and bloated on a few hundred unnecessary calories.

Drink from a glass. Pour your beer into a glass or mug to let some of the carbonation disperse. You won't get that bloated feeling as quickly as you would have if you'd drunk from the bottle.

Train your waiter. Order beer by the glass, not the pitcher; you'll probably drink less.

Slow down the stein way. Those hinged lids on German beer steins aren't just for show. They keep the beer fresh for leisurely drinking.

Do not challenge John Goodman to a drinking contest. With few exceptions, there's no way a 150-pounder can go one-on-one with a 250-pound drinker and wake up the winner. So scale down your drinks. To come out even, the 150-pounder can handle about half the alcohol of the 250-pounder.

Play the percentages. No-alcohol beers actually have a small percentage of alcohol, under 0.5 percent by law, compared to 4 percent content for regular beer and 3 percent for light. If you want a beer that truly contains no alcohol, look for one labeled "alcohol free."

Be a jigger bug. Unless you're a bartender who can rely entirely upon eye when measuring hard liquor into a drink, use a shot glass or jigger. If you pour straight from bottle to glass, you'll probably put in too much.

Have a cool one, not a cold one. The British and Europeans trash us for drinking beer cold. There may be more than snobbery involved. The closer to room temperature beer is, the better you can smell the malt, hops and yeast as you hoist it. Chilling, on the other hand, takes your nose out of play and may lead to guzzling. Buy a good brand of beer and enjoy it on the room-temperature side of cold. About 45° to 50° is ideal for most brands.

Order ice. A martini on the rocks is less potent than one served straight up, where there's no ice to melt and water down the drink. A frozen margarita is less potent than one served on the rocks: There's more water in all the crushed ice.

Party smartly. At a party, follow each drink with a glass of mineral water or soda. You'll always have something in your hand to sip, but you'll be getting half the liquor and calories you otherwise would. No-calorie carbonated mineral water and lime looks just like a 170-calorie gin and tonic. You'll also counteract alcohol's dehydrating actions.

Eat, then drink. Drinking only on a full stomach is "probably the single best thing you can do, besides drinking less, to reduce the severity of a hangover," says Mack Mitchell, M.D., vice-president of the Alcoholic Beverage Medical Research Foundation. "Food slows the absorption of alcohol, and the slower you absorb it, the less alcohol actually reaches the brain." The kind of food you eat doesn't matter much.

Scream not for ice cream. Latest drink to avoid: The hummer—rum, Kahlua and vodka, thrown into a blender with Häagen-Dazs. You hardly taste the alcohol when you blend it with ice cream. Also, you'll get fat while you're getting drunk: A pint of Häagen-Dazs used this way makes only three or four drinks. If you start seeing pink elephants, it may be your own expanding trunk.

Clear the air. Avoid smoky bars. A substance called acetaldehyde is found in alcohol *and* tobacco smoke, and it can make a bad hangover worse. There are now bars for folks who like to drink smoke free. One in New York is called Nosmo King.

Pass on the gas. Drinking bubbly beverages when you're drinking alcohol increases the rate at which alcohol is absorbed. Carbonation helps spread alcohol through the wall of your digestive tract, putting it into your bloodstream more quickly. Water or citrus juice is a better mixer than soda, again, particularly for preventing hangovers.

Bag the doggie. That image of a St. Bernard carrying brandy down the slopes to a half-frozen skier is medically slippery: Alcohol increases blood flow to the skin, giving you the immediate perception of warmth. But that heat is soon lost to the air, reducing your core body temperature. In short, alcohol makes you colder.

Say no to a nightcap. Alcohol makes for a poor sleeping potion because it disrupts sleep patterns. You may doze off initially, but in a few hours the effects will wear off and your body will slide into withdrawal, waking you up. If you have insomnia, avoid drinking at dinner and throughout the rest of the evening, suggests Michael Stevenson, Ph.D., a psychologist and sleep-disorders specialist in Mission Hills, California. Men who snore should also skip nightcaps: "Alcohol before bed makes snoring worse," says Earl V. Dunn, M.D., a Toronto sleep specialist.

Wine down the calories. "I have found I really appreciate a good glass of wine after a couple of days of abstention," James Suckling, senior editor of *The Wine Spectator,* has noticed. He's a fan of low-alcohol wines and has suggested switching from a full-bodied chardonnay (14 percent alcohol) to a traditional German Kabinett or Spatlese (10 percent or lower).

Watch your blood pressure. If you have high blood pressure, take it easy on the alcohol. A liquor cabinet full of studies has shown that heavier drinkers show greater increases in blood pressure and moderate drinkers show smaller increases. "Two drinks or fewer a day will probably have no detrimental effect on blood pressure, but when you go beyond that, you're looking for trouble," says Norman Kaplan, M.D., of the University of Texas Health Science Center at Dallas Southwestern Medical School. A heavy drinker with high blood pressure who stops altogether may see his pressure drop 10 to 25 points.

Protect your tummy. Heartburn or ulcer problems may flare up after you drink wine and beer. They make the stomach secrete more acids, further irritating the inner lining.

Prevent a bout with gout. If you suffer from gout, avoid alcohol, says Gary Stoehr, a University of Pittsburgh pharmacist. Alcohol seems to increase uric acid production, which can lead to gout attacks. Beer may be particularly undesirable because it is higher in a food substance called purine than wine or other spirits. If you drink, minimize your risk of a reaction by following this tip from Felix O. Kolb, M.D., of the University of California–San Francisco School of Medicine:

"Drink slowly and buffer wine with readily absorbed carbohydrates such as crackers, fruit and cheeses."

Try half-and-half. Order your cocktails with the alcohol on the side so you can mix your drink at your own pace. Pour half the shot into your mixer, and when that's gone, order another glass of mixer and add the rest of the alcohol.

Stay dry when you fly. Drinking on a flight ups your chances of suffering jet lag. "The cabin atmosphere contributes to dehydration," says Timothy Monk, Ph.D., a jet-lag specialist at the University of Pittsburgh. "Alcohol is a diuretic and will make you even drier. The best thing to do is drink fruit juice or decaffeinated soda."

Reason #4,763 not to drink and drive. A study by two Mississippi State University psychologists suggests moderate drinkers are even more likely than intoxicated ones to feel bold and self-assured about passing in the fast lane and driving at high speeds. Most people suffer some impairment of driving skills after only two drinks.

—Glenn Deutsch

Tripping Out Safely

*A hotel doctor who's seen it all offers advice
for the accident-prone tourist.*

••••••••••••••••••••••

MERELY *THINKING* ABOUT TRAVELING to a part of the world that has a warm climate, unspoiled beaches and friendly, easygoing people gives the average American abdominal cramps and the urge to run to the bathroom. Thoughts of exotic locations certainly affect my patients that way. I'm the house doctor of most of the hotels in Los Angeles—and the consequences of Mexican vacations contribute heavily to my income.

Patients stream in year-round, but mostly in late spring, asking for pills to prevent *turista*. Then they return from vacation begging me to cure it. I enjoy seeing these patients. I like any medical problem that I can help.

In the great scheme of things, traveler's diarrhea may not seem like much. But from my experience, even the most mundane illness or accident that wouldn't ruffle you at home can spoil your vacation more than discovering you'd never taken the lens cap off your camera.

Occasionally patients return with something more exotic than Montezuma's revenge. I can help them, too, although making the diagnosis can be tricky. Many of the illnesses and accidents that befall a traveler are preventable, and you can minimize the damage of other problems by following a few simple guidelines.

STOMACH TROUBLE, FIRST-CLASS

When the phone wakes me at 2:00 A.M., I can usually count on it being someone vomiting—the most common wee-hour symptom. When my beeper sounds as I'm jogging at 6:30 A.M., it's also a vomiter—one too polite to call earlier. I can usually help. But even if I can't, vomiting rarely lasts long, so guests give me the credit when they recover.

"The salad tasted funny" is a comment I might hear when I arrive at the victim's hotel room. Patients invariably blame an upset stomach on their previous meal. But unless they've been traveling in poor countries, they're usually wrong. In North America, Europe and other prosperous areas, a traveler's upset stomach is probably caused by a stomach flu caught from another person.

It's an easy mistake. The symptoms of a virus are the same as the symptoms of common food poisoning—nausea and vomiting, often with cramps and diarrhea—lasting about half a day, rarely more than a day.

If your symptoms last more than 24 hours, or if they're severe, call a doctor. If abdominal pain persists for more than 4 hours (especially if it's constant, rather than crampy), call a doctor. According to the textbooks, appendicitis consists of lower abdominal pain on the right side, with queasiness and perhaps some vomiting. But I've seen a surprising number of hotel guests with severe vomiting and generalized abdominal pain who ended up with an appendectomy—three during the two weeks it took to write this article. Something about travel must inflame the appendix.

While you're waiting out the symptoms, don't eat. Don't take drugs. Don't move. I'm always amazed at the fortitude of some victims. No sooner do they vomit than they rush to eat again, after which they rush back to the bathroom.

"I can't keep anything down," they tell me.

"Then why try?" I answer. "Your stomach is telling you something."

Putting anything into an irritable stomach makes it more irritable. Leave it in peace. Patients worry about getting dehydrated, but a day of vomiting won't harm a healthy adult (this is not so for infants and the elderly). Drink room-temperature, clear, nonalcoholic liquids such as water, chicken broth and ginger ale in sips, about six ounces or so hourly. Foods you can see "clear" through, such as Jell-O, are also good choices.

STOMACH TROUBLE, BUDGET-CLASS

Since the incubation period of Montezuma's revenge is generally three or four days, those who spend a week south of the border tend to get sick on the flight home or soon after checking into the hotel.

Vomiting occurs, but rarely is it enough to generate late-night calls; cramps and diarrhea are much worse. Victims worry about dysentery, amoebas and exotic parasites, but an ordinary germ causes almost all traveler's diarrhea. Called *Escherichia coli,* it lives peacefully in the human colon. Life in a poor country is a struggle for germs as well as humans, however, so foreign strains of *E. coli* defend themselves with an unpleasant toxin that inflames colons not accustomed to it.

Unlike rich-country stomach upsets, traveler's diarrhea is preventable and easy to cure. Although travel guides warn you to avoid tap water, ice, ice cream, unpasteurized dairy products and raw food except fruit that you've peeled yourself, these precautions may not work. Surveys of thousands of tourists reveal that those who avoid raw food and stay in the best hotels get sick as often as those who slurp down raw oysters and stay in budget lodgings. But food surveys are notoriously inaccurate, so it's still a good idea to avoid all these foods.

Your chance of getting sick is about one in four, but you can reduce this to one in ten by taking either an antibiotic daily or two bismuth subsalicylate tablets (such as Pepto-Bismol) four times a day. I prefer the bismuth-tablet solution to antibiotics. I think it's a bad idea to take antibiotics to *prevent* a disease, especially one that most travelers don't get, lasts only three or four days and is never fatal.

Treating traveler's diarrhea with antibiotics is another matter. Several work; the most common is sulfamethoxazole/trimethoprim, one tablet twice a day for five days. It's sensible to take along one complete course of therapy for each person on your trip. Many doctors, including me, are willing to prescribe it in advance.

But don't be in a hurry to use the antibiotic. Too many of my hotel guests felt a few cramps and quickly swallowed a pill or two. The cramps faded, and the guest decided that it wasn't the real thing and stopped taking the pills. Unfortunately, there weren't enough pills left to treat the full-blown attack that came later.

What I recommend is that travelers buy the over-the-counter diarrhea remedy loperamide. Use it for the first eight hours of any attack of diarrhea. If you're not better, begin the antibiotic—and finish it no matter how quickly you recover.

• •

Life's a Beach

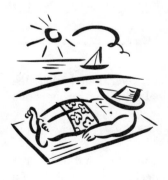

If you're one of those men who could never master a mantra, don't feel left out. A day at the beach or an afternoon sacked out on the couch can reduce stress just as much as meditation, according to a report by the National Academy of Sciences. The researchers said they could find no evidence meditation reduces stress and anxiety any better than simply resting quietly, or that it helped people cope with stress any better than "going to the beach or simply vegging out."

• •

TRAVELER'S ADVISORY

Here are several precautions experts recommend you take when traveling in an underdeveloped country.

Don't go barefoot. The soil teems with hookworms, which penetrate the skin and migrate to the intestine, where they attach and live off blood.

Don't go near the (fresh) water. If you swim or wade in fresh water, you can catch *schistosomiasis,* an infestation of a small worm that causes liver, kidney and bladder disease. The risks from salt water are no different from those on American beaches, but don't handle anything you can't identify, dead or alive. The barbs of a dead jellyfish can still sting.

Don't expose yourself to blood. This includes any blood product, such as gamma globulin or a vaccine. Avoid all injections because needles are often reused (this includes acupuncture treatments, tattooing and ear piercing). Make sure you can prove that you've had the required shots before traveling to an underdeveloped country. Otherwise you might be forced to have them at the airport. Avoiding blood products helps protect you from AIDS—a real risk in Haiti and in parts of Africa—and hepatitis. Needless to say, unprotected sex is foolish in any part of the world.

Don't buy medicines. This warning includes all countries outside of North America and western Europe. Most nations don't have a Food and Drug Administration (FDA) as strict as ours, and I'm regularly amazed by medications hotel guests pick up on their trips—drugs turned down by the FDA or taken off the market for toxicity.

• •

Look for these danger signs: high fever, bloody diarrhea and persistent (not crampy) abdominal pain. They're signs of a more serious infection.

IN-FLIGHT EARACHES

If your ears hurt when the plane takes off and feel worse when it's landing, that's not an ear infection. But it's also not a welcome experience so early in your trip. Most likely you have a mild cold or allergy, and swelling of your nasal lining has blocked the tubes that link your middle ear with the outside. During changes in cabin pressure, air trapped in your clogged ears expands and contracts, stretching the eardrums painfully.

Airline personnel are surprisingly unhelpful. (I treat their earaches, too.) They cheerfully advise passengers to chew gum or to pinch their noses and swallow, maneuvers useful for only the mildest obstruction. The best preventive is a strong nasal decongestant spray. Before takeoff, spray both nostrils thoroughly, wait five minutes, then repeat. Tilt your head to the side and sniff the spray deeply into your nose. Do the same before the plane begins its descent. An oral decongestant helps, but not as well as a spray.

Even a spray isn't foolproof. Sometimes it doesn't work, and discomfort can last for days. See a doctor if you're too uncomfortable. I make sure an infection isn't present (it's rare) and hand out painkilling eardrops.

Don't be surprised if your doctor prescribes antibiotics. Your eardrums will look quite red after having been stretched for days. It's easy to mistake that for an infection. In this case, the antibiotics won't help. When you do see a doctor, be sure to tell him or her that you have recently flown while suffering from a cold or allergy. Look for these danger signs: If the pain disappears and you notice fluid in the ear, the drum has probably perforated. This is less catastrophic than it sounds because most perforations heal, but a doctor should examine you. And naturally, you shouldn't fly if you already have ear pain.

BUG BITES

Foreign bugs are less exotic than you think. Just about anywhere you go, mosquitoes bother you the most. To keep them—and most other insects—away, take plenty of insect repellent containing diethyltoluamide (deet).

Guests are often alarmed when small, itchy pimples appear on their legs. When I diagnose flea bites, victims usually protest that no one else in the room was bothered. But that's because people vary greatly in their sensitivity to the bites. Flea bites may leave a permanent brown stain when they heal, so make sure to apply repellent to your vulnerable legs and feet.

Although most ticks are harmless, they can spread diseases, such as typhus, Rocky Mountain spotted fever and Lyme disease. Removing a tick as soon as possible decreases your chance of infection. Ignore most tick-removal advice you've heard. Don't paint the tick with gasoline, lighter fluid or petroleum jelly, and don't torment it with an ice cube, burning cigarette or hot nail. The best way to remove a tick is to pull it out. Grasp it near the skin with tweezers and pull backward. Exert slow, steady pressure backward, taking five to ten seconds to pull it off. Despite terrible warnings about allowing the head to break off and stay in the skin, no great harm results. Leave it alone. After removing the tick, dab the area with an antiseptic or an antimicrobial cream.

Important: Save the tick, dead or alive, in a jar marked with the date and location of the bite. Keep it for six to eight weeks. If you develop symptoms of Lyme disease (a bull's-eye rash over the bite, flulike fatigue, chills or muscle aches), take the tick to your doctor for identification.

SLIPS AND SLICES

Getting off the tour bus at the end of the day, a traveler stumbles and twists his ankle painfully. His wife rushes him to the local hospital, where, after waiting three hours in the emergency room, they're relieved to learn that he hasn't broken anything. He returns to the hotel with a bottle of painkillers and the ankle securely wrapped.

He could have stayed in bed. While an injury can certainly upset your travel plans, most injuries are less serious than they seem. If this happens to you, apply ice to keep down the swelling, collect your thoughts and phone a doctor.

"But what if it's fractured?" guests ask when I suggest waiting a day or two. The answer is that there's no urgency about fractures of the toes, feet, ankles, fingers, hands, wrists, arms and nose. Even if a cast is required, a doctor must wait for the swelling to go down. The exception to this no-urgency rule is this: If there's severe pain unrelieved by rest, elevation or over-the-counter pain relievers, or there's blood, protruding bone or shortness of breath, seek medical attention immediately.

Of course, possible fractures of large bones, such as the pelvis, hips, spine or skull, should not wait.

Cuts, unless they're serious, usually don't require a trip to an emergency room either. For small wounds, suturing is less important than people believe. It's a cosmetic procedure that pulls wound edges together to make a thinner scar. If you

• •

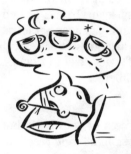

Get All the Z's You Need

In a Gallup Poll of Americans, one-third complained that they woke up in the middle of the night and couldn't get back to sleep. Are *you* a member of this fraternity of the fatigued? If so, try some of these sleep aids.

Stay on the same sleep schedule seven days a week. Sleeping late on weekends can screw up your natural sleep patterns.

Don't be afraid of the dark. Morning's first light may be waking you too early. Use drapes or heavy shades to darken your bedroom.

Don't waste time in bed. There's no use "trying" to sleep—it's guaranteed to keep you awake. If you can't snooze, get out of bed and do something pleasantly monotonous like watching TV.

Watch what you drink. Coffee as early as 4:00 P.M. can keep you awake at bedtime. Colas and chocolate also contain caffeine.

Take a bath. Several studies have shown that a warm bath four or five hours before bedtime can help you sleep.

Walk yourself to sleep. Don't exercise vigorously just before bed. A short evening walk, however, can help relax you.

Have more sex. Researchers have found that hormones triggered during sex can enhance sleep in some people.

Insomnia has a number of causes, among them stress, diet, medications, illness and breathing problems. If you can't easily fall asleep or stay asleep throughout the night for a month or so at a time, talk to your doctor.

don't mind a small scar, and the cut is shallow, clean it with soap and water and bring the edges together with a Band-Aid. If you're in doubt, speak to a doctor.

Injured tendons, nerves and arteries must be repaired. See a doctor for a deep cut where there's a chance that these are damaged. A wound must be closed within 8 to 12 hours. After this period, suturing is not a good idea—it traps too many germs inside, so most doctors leave it open to heal.

Is it easy to find a doctor when you're on a trip? Usually. Overseas, call the American Embassy/Consulate for the name and number of an English-speaking physician. In the United States, ask the concierge or the on-duty manager for a referral to a physician. Or ask for the name and location of the nearest hospital emergency room; if you're really sick, call 911 or the appropriate local emergency service number.

SKIN PROBLEMS

If you erupt into itchy welts over most of your body but otherwise feel well, that's probably hives, an allergic reaction. When seeing a hotel guest, I ask about new drugs, foods or lotions, and most often the victim simply shakes his head. Patients get upset when I can't pinpoint the cause, so I explain that hives frequently appear mysteriously. Unless they recur, the cause remains obscure. No treatment shortens the attack, which may last several days, but an over-the-counter antihistamine can suppress itching.

Most patients believe that a patch of dry, itchy skin is ringworm. If it is ringworm, applying an over-the-counter antifungal cream may help. But large itchy areas, particularly if you're middle-aged or older, are probably excessively dry skin, so any ointment works fine.

Apply cortisone cream. Cortisone doesn't cure anything, but it makes everything feel better because it suppresses the body's inflammatory response. When skin is damaged, the inflammatory response makes blood rush to the area, which then turns red. Fluid, blood cells and certain body chemicals pour into the skin, producing itching and burning. Although this response is essential to repair an injury or kill invading organisms, it's just a nuisance when provoked by an allergy, dryness or minor irritation.

•••

PACK A HEALTH KIT

If you're traveling to a foreign country, consider taking along a kit bag containing the following items.

- Adhesive strips
- Gauze pads and cotton swabs
- Elastic bandage
- Pain pills (aspirin, acetaminophen or ibuprofen)
- Diarrhea remedies (loperamide or bismuth tablets)
- Nasal decongestant sprays
- Antihistamines
- Motion-sickness remedies
- ½ percent hydrocortisone cream for allergic rashes
- Antifungal cream
- Zinc oxide, petroleum jelly, calamine lotion
- Sunscreen
- Tweezers, scissors, safety pins
- Oil of cloves—an anesthetic for a painful tooth

If your doctor is willing, ask for the following items.

- A treatment for *turista:* five days' worth of sulfamethoxazole/trimethoprim
- A motion-sickness remedy in a skin patch
- A strong antinauseant: prochlorperazine

•••

The fact that cortisone prevents inflammation means that it can delay healing and suppress the body's defense against infections. The weak concentrations now available without a prescription, however, are not likely to do any harm. I would caution against using a prescription cortisone cream, which contains a more substantial dose, without an accurate diagnosis by a physician.

THE DRAG OF JET LAG

If you're crossing time zones, force yourself to stay awake until the new bedtime when you arrive at your destination. You'll think the worst is over when you finally fall into bed, but count on waking up sometime in the early morning hours. If you're someplace where your internal clock says it's time to get up and it's actually bedtime there, lie quietly in bed. Relax and think pleasant thoughts until morning. Then get up and expose yourself to bright light. This helps reset your body clock to the new cycle of light and dark.

In a day or two your sleep cycle should adjust. Plan vigorous activities, such as walking tours, during the first few days; don't go to plays or other events where drowsiness could ruin the fun.

—Michael Oppenheim, M.D.

Part 4

MAN-TO-MAN
TALK

Go Ahead,
Make My Day

There's a part of us always itching for a fight.
Maybe that's why Steven Seagal gets millions
while Alan Alda gets forgotten?

●●●●●●●●●●●●●●●●●●●●●●

THE FIRST TIME I realized I was capable of murdering someone, I was 15. A novice surfer hazed by the older boys, I let one of them help me carry my new surfboard (long and heavy in those days) up the concrete stairs from the beach. He lifted the tail, then purposely dropped it on the concrete, crunching the fiberglass. He laughed. I lunged, and it took three others to untangle the sandy knot of our bodies. I'd grown up in a family where it was rare even to raise one's voice in anger, but that day I discovered how easy it is to sink into the fire below thought. It felt good.

This admission does not come easily; perhaps more than the average guy, I've struggled to maintain a nonviolent outlook. During the Vietnam War, I was a conscientious objector. Later I lived for two years in a yoga ashram. And recently I've spent a number of Sundays sitting quietly with the Quakers, listening to messages of peace.

But I'm still a man, and though I may cuddle with my sons, listen to Andreas Vollenweider tapes and support disarmament, there will always be a primitive core that, far from fleeing violence, revels in it.

It's just not the same for women. Males of all ages in virtually every culture are more physically aggressive than females, says psychiatrist and anthropologist Melvin Konner, M.D., Ph.D., of Emory University. Males also exceed females in risk taking and thrill seeking.

MALES ARE NATURAL HUNTERS

"Natural selection prepared men to be hunters, and we've departed from that role only in the past 10,000 years, a short time in evolutionary terms," Dr. Konner says. "We are, in effect, hunters in business suits."

Perhaps that's one reason why, in the United States alone, more than 400 people are slain each week, most of them by men. Feminists may joke about "testosterone poisoning," but the fact is that this male hormone does play a strong role in aggression. Indeed, convicts serving time for violent crimes tend to have higher testosterone levels than nonviolent inmates, according to studies at Georgia State University.

This raises a question: If aggression is part of our makeup, how do we open ourselves to it without doing something violent?

Sports provide a venerable answer. What better way to satisfy aggressive urges than to smash a tennis ball or, even better, slam into your opponent on the football field?

"Extreme aggression, competition, domination. I enjoy getting into that mode," confesses Russ Frydenborg, a biologist with the Florida Department of Environmental Regulation and an avid member of the Florida State University Water Polo Club. "It's hard to describe why it's so much fun to kick ass. You're driving toward the goal to score and your heart is pounding like a hammer and someone grabs your legs and you just kick him in the face."

In fact, sports not only vent aggression, they can also draw it out of otherwise mild-mannered men. A study of the Harvard wrestling team showed a rise in testosterone levels during matches, with winners posting a significantly larger rise than losers. A similar study at the University of Nebraska measured a hormonal jump for victors and slump for losers among tennis players.

But a man doesn't even have to be an active participant to let loose. Spectators, in a stadium crowd or in the comfort of their own living rooms, can get their ya-yas out by shouting obscenities, or death threats, at offending players and referees.

AGGRESSION FEELS GOOD

"Pleasure as a motive for aggression is universal," writes the German naturalist Irenaus Eibl-Eibesfeldt, Ph.D., in his work *Love and Hate*. The buildup of aggression causes an unpleasant tension, he says, and releasing it feels good.

Even in the peaceful halls of academia, researchers were able to measure just how good it feels to get mad, then get even. Students were intentionally harassed while they tried to solve certain problems, their slow burn causing a rise in blood pressure. The angry subjects were then told that the experimenter, the source of their suffering, would solve the problem himself and they could press a button whenever he made a mistake. Some subjects were led to believe the button delivered electric shocks, others that it merely switched on a signal light. Blood pressure quickly dropped in those who believed they were zapping the tyrant in the lab coat, but the others stayed hot, and their blood pressure remained high.

Certainly the joy of vengeance has not been lost on Hollywood. Most violent films follow a standard plot: The bad guy humiliates, injures or kills the good guy's wife (or girl-friend, child or pet); then, at the climax, the good guy (with whom you identify till the veins pop out in your neck) gets to rupture the punk's spleen in slow motion.

Schwarzenegger, Stallone and, more recently, Steven Seagal have made millions for themselves playing characters who snap bones, kick solar plexuses and fire heavy artillery at slimy villains.

Unfortunately, shown to the wrong audience at the wrong time, such shoot-'em-ups may very well fan the flames of aggression rather than put out the fire. Aggressive feelings, once aroused in the spectator, aren't always worked off—which may partly explain the fights stirred up in theaters showing movies like *Colors* and *Boyz N the Hood*.

Apart from attacking an innocent bystander, however, experts agree that the worst approach to aggression is to repress it.

"I see patients with headaches, ulcers and heart problems who haven't discovered yet that they are furious," says Herbert Strean, Ph.D., a psychoanalyst and coauthor of *Our Wish to Kill*.

LET IT OUT—OR ELSE!

Besides squeezing your chest and burning a hole in your gut, lugging around pent-up aggression often merely delays the inevitable: a violent outburst that can have disastrous consequences.

Of course, natural aggression is only one factor in male rage. Everyday frustrations and indignities add to it. And for those who've grown up in dysfunctional families, anger can become a way of life.

"Many of us are carrying a residue of abuse from our childhoods," says psychotherapist Marvin Allen, director of the Texas Men's Institute in San Antonio. "We end up project-ing our anger onto others, turning our bosses into our fathers, our wives into our mothers, coworkers into rival siblings and so forth.

"I work with men who say, 'I can't let myself get angry because if I ever do, I'm liable to tear this office down; I'll kill somebody.' I hand them a plastic bat and give them permission to fly into a rage, scream and cuss and beat the stuffing out of a pillow. And with a focused outlet for their rage, they do fine."

Allen advises thinking of anger as information. If you're angry, your job is to communicate that fact plus tell why you're angry. That way, you not only release anger but also take a step toward solving the problem at hand. This is especially important if you're dealing with someone you love. You might say, "I'm really pissed. I love you and I'm not going to leave you, but *damn* it makes me angry when you do that!"

FEEL THE EMOTION

Common sense tells us to put aside our anger at times. However much we may want to, we can't always pipe up and tell the boss where to go. That's called *suppression,* Allen says, and it's not necessarily bad. *Repressing* anger, on the other hand, means you don't even recognize that you're angry because you can't allow yourself to feel that emotion.

"The boss throws work on your desk at 4:30 and tells you to get it out by morning. You contain your anger for the moment, but you know you're angry and you know its source. Then you can go home and gripe about it. But if you don't even acknowledge anger, you just get irritable. Then you go

• •

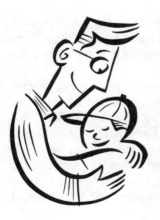

Dads: Hug Your Kids
Hugs and physical affection with parents strongly predict successful friendships, marriages and careers in a child's future, says a 36-year study published in the *Journal of Personality and Social Psychology.* Seventy percent of the kids with affectionate parents did well for themselves socially, compared with only 30 percent of the kids with cold-fish parents, and Dad's hugs were found to be as important as Mom's.

• •

MARTIAL AARRGGHH!

One constructive way of harnessing aggression might be through the discipline of a martial art, according to Richard Carrera, Ph.D., a University of Miami psychologist. He studied male karate students and found that, compared with other men, the martial artists were better able to turn their aggression on or off.

"Karate devalues impulsive violence," Dr. Carrera explains, "and because of its emphasis on discipline, it tends to increase one's self-control." He also noted that karate boosted men's confidence that they could handle themselves in an aggressive situation. "Whenever you increase a person's security, you lower the likelihood that he'll act out violently. Violence is usually the resort of somebody who is frightened or who has low self-esteem."

• •

home and take out your anger on your wife and children without realizing what you're doing."

For some men, however, talking things out will just not be enough. That's why societies have traditionally provided dangerous but potentially redeeming alternatives to antisocial violence.

A boy with strong aggressive and risk-taking traits could grow up to be a terrific cop, for example, instead of a terrible thug, Strean says. It all depends on how his parents, peers and neighborhood sway him.

In wartime, of course, aggression is prized and praised. Thus, a hard-hitting soldier who charges a machine-gun nest and single-handedly wipes out the enemy is honored as a life-saving hero.

"Giving young male delinquents a choice of going to jail or going to Vietnam made some sense," says San Diego–based Warren Farrell, Ph.D., author of *Why Men Are the Way They Are*. "The same trait that got them into trouble—bold aggression in the face of danger—may well make them heroes in combat. The hero then gets decorated instead of incarcerated."

But whether we're warriors on Wall Street or rifle-toting soldiers, the problem of male aggression remains universal.

Few scientists would claim that our genes and hormones condemn us to violence or war, but many believe that our *capacity* for violence can never be erased.

Sometimes I wonder: If I could transport my adult consciousness back into my 15-year-old body and relive that surfboard incident, how would I react now? Well, perhaps I wouldn't try to murder my persecutor or even cause him permanent injury. But I'd still try my best to beat the hell out of him. Why? Because he asked for it, and I'm a man, and it would have been murder for me to go through life without the satisfaction of knowing that, when it really mattered to me, justice was done.

—Mark Canter

Do It Your Way

It's okay to live your life in a manly kind of way. A psychiatrist says being proud of manhood could save you.

• •

PARDON OUR TESTOSTERONE, ladies, but a guy's got to be what he's got to be. "Men need to live their lives—the ups and the downs—in a *male* way," says psychiatrist Kenneth Wetcher, M.D. "And if they need to reach out for help, that whole process has to happen in a male way, too, or it won't work."

Much of psychotherapy, however, is skewed toward women's needs, says Dr. Wetcher. Men are expected to bare their deepest feelings, something most are well trained *not* to do.

"Women catch on quickly because they're experts at emoting," he says. "But most guys are expert at stowing their feelings. So when a therapist demands that a man spill his guts, it's often too hard for him and he drops out."

Two years ago the Houston-based psychiatrist founded Men's Forum, a therapy group that deals with problems in a male context. "We start by talking," he explains. "We discuss ways in which men have been trained to function: as husband, father, son, brother, friend, employee, boss. Then we attach feelings to those roles. For example, as a husband, you may feel obligation, desire, jealousy, loneliness, pride. Gradually, the men begin connecting with and expressing their emotions."

Men's Health asked Dr. Wetcher to share some of what he's learned.

Q. You've said therapists must consider not just the problem—such as job stress or divorce—but the specific ways men might react to the problem. What would be a typical male reaction and how does it differ from a woman's?

A. Men are much more likely to resort to rage and aggression. It's considered an acceptable way for men to cope with feeling out of control. You'll hear about a man breaking his hand by slugging a wall with his fist, but you won't hear about a woman working out her frustrations that way.

Another example would be a guy beating up his ex-wife's new boyfriend rather than working on his own pain of loss. Since anger is permitted, any strong emotion that is not permitted is converted into anger.

Men need to step back a moment and see if anger is really what they're feeling. The trouble is, we've been trained not to hurt. In sports the coach tells you to *play with the pain*. And if you don't want to be humiliated, you learn that early.

Q. Why are we trained to use anger that way?

A. Anger and aggression often help us compete against other men, on the football field, on the battlefield or in business. When we step outside the ring, however, it's suddenly not okay to be combative. You can't yell at the cop who just pulled you over. It gets confusing.

I have a client who is a Vietnam vet and works at one of the oil companies here. He was functioning reasonably well, when one day there was an explosion on the work site. He saw a bunch of his buddies lying in pieces. He flashed back to what happened in the war, and he felt like going berserk. He wanted to kick down the supervisor's door and break furniture over the guy's head. It was tough to accept that acting out his rage against the "enemy" was no longer allowed. Men like that often turn to drugs or alcohol to subdue themselves.

Q. What are some other uniquely male problems that we should be on the lookout for?

A. Some guys believe they must always succeed and that failure of any sort reflects badly on them. A woman can fail to pry off a pickle-jar lid and not make a big deal out of it. But if her husband can't open it, he'll get a hernia trying. He's embarrassed. That's a mistake. We all fail frequently, and you can't succeed without extending yourself enough to risk failure. Men seem to understand that on the playing field, but they don't carry it into their daily lives.

Related to that is a reluctance to seek help. Men believe they're supposed to solve all their problems on their own. A guy will pay big money to have a pro help him with his golf swing or tennis game or to have an expert take care of his car, but with physical or emotional problems, he tries to tough it out. Three times as many men as women abuse drugs and alcohol—because they don't know how to cope with their feelings—and yet three times as many women seek help for substance abuse.

Q. Are you saying that the traditional male upbringing is harmful?

A. I want to get away from the apologists who say we need to atone for our sins by becoming more like women. That would be unfortunate in the same way that the assimilation of ethnic groups in our country or the loss of accents is unfortunate—everyone trying to speak like a Midwesterner.

The bottom line is, the differences in the way the sexes behave aren't just learned. Our psyches really are distinct in hard-wired, physiological ways. For example, men are generally better at looking at details and working on different tasks at the same time: The husband is reading the paper and watching TV as his wife talks to him and she says, "You haven't heard a word I've said"; then he repeats her lines verbatim. Women generally are better at looking at the big picture, so they often understand relationships faster or better than men do. These are due to biological differences in the brain.

Q. Can you describe another distinctly male reaction to stressful situations?

A. Withdrawal—retreating into silence—is a common male coping strategy. Or becoming obsessive about work or hobbies or money. But being a workaholic isn't only an avoidance tactic, as some psychologists would have us believe. For example, a man who wants to earn his wife's love might choose to work overtime to provide things for her.

Q. Still, it doesn't sound like you think that would be a very good way to win her love.

A. Things get particularly confusing when you get into relationships. Men don't realize that there is often a difference between what women say they want in a man and what they really do want. Most women will say they want a warm, open, loving kind of man, but in fact, they often pursue just the other kind: the man who has the greatest potential to be successful, the one who's willing to work overtime. In our modern business environment, that's probably not going to be the guy who's most sensitive.

Q. What are some other ways men and women are different?

A. Men seem to have internal time limits. When couples have arguments, the woman often doesn't want to stop until the issue is resolved, whereas the man at some point will say, "I've had enough. Let's stop now and continue later" or "I don't want to talk about it here." Women more often insist that the argument get finished now—even if it's taking place in the first-class cabin of a jumbo jet.

Q. Men are often accused by women of being afraid of commitment. Are we guilty as a group?

A. Commitment boggles a lot of guys. We see it as ownership, and we don't want to feel like we're owned. So we never give ourselves a chance to develop a satisfying relationship or to clarify for the woman what commitment means to us.

Then again, many of us put all our eggs in one basket—such as identifying totally with our work roles. We become one-dimensional. Aside from being, say, a well-paid lawyer, we're nothing. This applies to relationships, too. Your girlfriend or wife becomes the only person in the world you share your life with, so if you break up, your life is on hold—until your next girlfriend.

Women tend to have women friends that they are close to. So they have human contact and sharing outside of a love relationship.

Q. We've heard it said for years that men should have more male friends. Is there any other place to look for companionship outside of love and marriage?

A. Too many men make the mistake of not getting close to their sons, usually because their fathers never got close to them. Fathers need to make a special effort to be intimate with their kids.

And I think a lot of men miss out on the satisfaction of being mentors. There is so much pressure to focus on yourself and your own success that you frequently don't take the time to find a young person at work who could benefit from your experience. Mentoring is an ancient and noble role that we are skipping altogether.

Q. Should men and women parent differently?

A. Maybe we should skip the word *parenting* and call it *fathering* and *mothering* because, again, there really are distinctions, whether the differences are learned or biological. Yet when we think about fathers taking care of their children, our model tends to be mothering. A movie like *Mr. Mom.* That's not fathering; that's mothering.

Generally, women have been trained and, I think, have the superior biology for nurturing and caring. Men, on the other hand, are much better at coaching—that is, giving kids the slack to get themselves into a bit of trouble and then providing the pointers to get themselves out of trouble.

Once we had a group session where a man needed to bring his eight-month-old daughter. When his wife arrived to pick her up, everyone noticed the difference in the way they related to the girl. Dad would swing her by her legs and let her crawl around the floor and drool on everyone's shoes. The wife cringed. Her impulse was to run and pick the kid up to protect her from the wrath of strangers.

It's great for a child to know that one parent will expose him to some risks and let him learn his own lessons, and the other parent is going to rush to kiss the boo-boo if he gets hurt. It's difficult for one parent to be good at both these things, plus it's confusing to the child.

Q. Is there anything short of therapy that can help a guy feel better about being a man these days? Couldn't just being on a men's softball team allow him to work on issues of male friendships?

A. Possibly. But generally, men will focus on the activity and not on sharing their feelings. Women, when they play together on a team, develop some self-disclosure and intimacy. So men usually need to take a conscious step, and that is best done by getting involved in a group made for that. It doesn't have to be formal therapy: Nowadays in most cities, men are getting together in what are often called men's support groups. Then you can export that sensitivity to your other relationships.

—Mark Canter

You Can Win

Arguing is as fundamental to school-yard basketball as the dribble. If you can't master the fine art of arguing, you can't win.

•••••••••••••••••••••

A DAYDREAM: I HAVE THE BALL. I beat my man to the baseline and glide to the basket. Weakside help arrives. I raise my dribble and lift the two defenders off the ground. Airborne sentinels, they hover above, denying access to the rim. I take off an instant later, floating past their useless barricade to the other side of the hoop. I flip the ball into the basket and drift back to earth, reveling in the perfection of the moment.

But in my daydream there is always a bitter epilogue. I hear the wail of a human voice. "No. No. No." The defensive man I beat on the baseline is pointing to an imaginary footprint on the cement. "You stepped on the line. No basket. Our ball." As always, my masterful flight has ended in the dust with petty mortals. And the bickering must begin.

Arguing is as fundamental to school-yard basketball as the dribble. In the school yard there are no clocks and no referees. There are infinite possibilities for infraction and the decisions are in the hands of the contestants.

Simply put, if you can't or won't defend yourself verbally in a top-of-the-line school-yard game, the game I play in New York and that is played in every city in America, you won't win.

I haven't always played this way. Twenty years ago I played small-forward in the Ivy League. I used to complain to the referee a lot. The refs ignored my complaints. It is not logic that wins basketball arguments. Especially in the school yard.

After graduation, I headed to the school yards of New York City to prove myself. As the years went by I lost a half a step, and then the other half. But as I slowed down I mastered the art of arguing on the basketball court.

One principle that allows the school-yard game to progress is the idea of "respecting" your opponent's call. No matter how outrageous, every call must, theoretically, be respected. If a bad call is made, an experienced player will allow the call and make a bad call of his own.

I have seen many games deteriorate into dreary exchanges of bad calls. Larry will make a bad call and Hollyroc will retaliate. The old guys are almost always behind lengthy standoffs; their legs are gone but not their wits. "I was hit," Hollyroc announces. "By who?" Larry wants to know. Hollyroc isn't careful and he points to the wrong man. Larry picks up the mistake. "No way. He wasn't near you. He didn't foul you, and you don't get the ball." Hollyroc leans against the fence. This is going to be a long one. The younger guys are frustrated. They mill around the court mumbling curses. They want to play. They want to block shots and dunk. The darkness deepens. Two voices duel in the shadows.

KEEP IT SIMPLE

The argument between the two men illustrates an important principle. Hollyroc got himself in trouble because he overextended his argument. He wasn't sure who fouled him, so he should have refused to be forced into identifying the perpetrator. By picking the wrong man he created a crack in what should have been an open-and-shut case. Larry picked up the flaw and hung his entire defense on it. When your call is righteous you don't let yourself be drawn into elaborating. You keep it simple.

I'm playing two-on-two at a half court along Columbus Avenue. An old college teammate is on my team. He's burying the jump shot and giving up the ball at just the right time. We're holding our own against two young whippets from uptown.

I know my friend—he came to win. Point game. The ball skips past the baseline. The kid guarding me calls for the ball. He points at my friend. "It hit your leg," he says.

"Bull," my friend snaps, and snatches the ball.

"I saw the ball hit your leg—you're lying," the kid insists.

"No way," my friend says as he inbounds the ball. I am six feet from the basket with my back to the hoop. I can feel the kid guarding me is mad. I step away for the fadeaway jump shot. I jerk my head and the kid rises like a puppet on a string. I step underneath and bank in the four-footer. We win.

The kid hasn't forgotten the call that cost him the game. "Why you gotta lie?" he asks my friend.

As we walk home I look at my buddy quizzically. "The ball hit your leg," I say. "I saw it."

"To hell with them," he answers. "They were punks. We were better. We deserved to win. Justice."

Justice, maybe, but not always truth. One of the ways to win a hoops argument is to lie.

SAVING UP FOR A BAD CALL

Some guys establish a reputation for honesty throughout the contest just so they can make a bad call when the game is on the line. "It's the first foul I've called," they'll whine. Don't fall for it.

At the school yard there's a fine line betewen ruining the game with bull and mastering the art of the argument. But master it you must. You can't be above it. They'll butcher you when you try to shoot and call touch fouls on you at the other end. Give up your call at the end of the game and nobody will want you on their team, no matter how good you are. Don't even consider being one of those Dudley Doright types who call fouls on themselves. "I hit you. Your ball." How obnoxious.

The school-yard basketball debater must exhibit a vast belief in himself. It's extremely bad form to appeal to observers on the sidelines to verify your call. You don't need support from the sidelines, and you don't need concurrence from your teammates. Make your call and stand by it.

I HATED TO DO IT

Only once did I give up a call. And I was happy do to it. It was on a July 4th about 15 years ago. Anybody who had any sense was at the beach. I was at West 4th Street, and a sparse crowd had gathered around the fence. A guy with bowlegs was guarding me. I later found out it was Charlie Yelverton, who was to have a season at Fordham that winter that would make his coach, Digger Phelps, a famous man. A 6-foot-3 forward, he was too small for the NBA but he could hop with anybody. On that day in the Village he bounded around the court and hovered around the rim like a hummingbird. I hit two jump shots and he came out to guard me. I faked the shot and he rocketed into space. I took note of his sneakers dangling above my waist as I put the ball on the ground and drove to the basket. I took off for a lay-up but by the time I put the ball up, Yelverton was back. I am not sure how he did it, but he rose over my left shoulder and hijacked my shot just as it began its descent to the basket. What I had witnessed was amazing. But it was also a clear case of goaltending. I hated to make the call, but I did. "Goaltending," I screamed.

The upper-echelon school-yard players don't like to call goaltending. Leaping ability is so prized that such a call is considered mean-spirited and petty. But I was young then, and goaltending it was. The small group of connoisseurs on the fence groaned at my indiscretion. Play was halted. My teammates were silent. Yelverton walked over to me. I turned away. I didn't want to hear any crap. The ball was on its way down. But he spoke softly. "Listen," he said. "We're both leapers. Why would you want to make a call like that?" Both leapers? The idea was immensely appealing to me. I spun around and faced the other players. "False call," I declared in a landmark decision.

Since that day I have never called goaltending on anybody. I may have mastered the art of arguing to cover up the yawning holes in my game. But I have my pride.

—*Greg Donaldson*

Lost in Splitsville

Divorce can be a lonely place, full of anxiety, uncertainty and self-doubt. But picking up the pieces after the lawyers leave is possible.

• •

THE MAN HAD BEEN a prisoner of war in Vietnam. He'd suffered unspeakable fear, pain and degradation. But as awful as that experience was, the man told his psychologist, he had recently confronted something even worse: a divorce.

"In prison I could take the physical pain. I lived eight years on crutches because I broke my right leg when I bailed out. I was tortured and I found I could stand that. But the emotional test of the past few weeks has been hard to pass," the man told *Men's Health* advisor Herb Goldberg, Ph.D.

Not every man gets whacked that badly by a divorce. But nobody emerges from the experience unscathed or unchanged. Life is not one big party after your average marriage breaks up. Splitsville can be a lonely place, full of anxiety, uncertainty and self-doubt. Getting past all that takes time.

"My divorce is like a cold I can't quite shake," says Bill Miller (name changed), a Los Angeles public relations executive. "It's been two years and I feel it less nowadays, but it lingers on in my life."

Clinical psychologist Judith Wallerstein, Ph.D., who studied 60 divorced couples for her book *Second Chances*, found that ten years after divorce, half the men had serious misgivings about their decision to divorce. "Many surveys have found that it takes two or three years for both men and women to get their lives back together," she adds. Some had trouble concentrating on their work for up to two years after a split.

ROUGH GOING

What's the message? That it's easier to stay in a lousy marriage than to face the pain of divorce? No. In fact, studies have shown that it's probably healthier in the long run to get a divorce than to stay in an insufferable relationship. Still, very few men can walk away from a bad marriage and step directly into the good life. You've got to expect that the terrain is going to be difficult, both physically and emotionally.

"Even with my training and experience as a professional counselor, I wasn't prepared for the emotional impact of divorce when it hit me," admits San Francisco psychologist Mel Krantzler, Ph.D.

Mind you, Dr. Krantzler, who went on to create a series of divorce-recovery workshops and to author *Creative Divorce*, isn't all doom and gloom: "It's up to the man what he makes of it. The consequences can be negative. They can also be very positive."

No matter what your attitude toward the proceedings, handling the day-to-day emotional baggage is hard work. Recently divorced or separated men frequently describe the way they feel in terms like "I feel suspended between the past and the future," "I'm nervous because I don't know what's in store for me in the next year," and "Despite the breakup I still feel a sense of attachment to my ex-wife."

Just about every man will go through a period of mourning following a divorce, even if he and his wife had been separated for some time. Feelings of guilt—especially if he did the leaving—and failure are normal. "Divorce is like a death in the family," says psychologist Myrna Hartley, Ph.D. "Even if you've ended up hating your wife, when the marriage ends, something important has died with it and you need to mourn its passing. It's painful to pass through this period, but you'll come out much stronger in the end."

ALLOW YOURSELF TO MOURN

Skip this stage—say, by being a wild man about town— and you're inviting long-term problems such as depression, warns University of Oklahoma psychologist Donald J. Bertoch, Ph.D. He recommends therapy, maintaining positive relationships with friends and family and basically refraining from making major decisions during the first postdivorce year.

The idea is to get through your grief without giving a bunch of it to your kids, family, boss, coworkers...and dates. "Finish the grief process before developing a new significant relationship," Dr. Bertoch says. "Otherwise, it will contaminate the quality of caring and loving for the other person."

One key to successful emotional recovery is to resist the urge to blame everything that went wrong on your ex-wife. Says famed divorce lawyer Melvin Belli in his book *Divorcing,* "If I had it to do all over again, here is how I would handle my own divorce: I would recognize that it takes two to make a marriage turn sour. That means that I have shared in the responsibility for my marriage ending. Not intentionally, but because I let things that were going wrong drift, and I believed everything that created arguments and tension was always the other person's fault."

Belli has had a lot of practice at this (he's been divorced four times), and he knows what he's talking about. Dr. Krantzler, who is co-author of Belli's book, agrees. "The problem may be that *you* have been dealing with interpersonal relationships unsuccessfully. Accept that and you'll find the remedies."

LEARN YOUR LESSON

"Divorce is an opportunity to learn the hard way how to relate to women," Dr. Krantzler adds. "It's also a place to set your priorities straight. Life's problems aren't solved by making money, owning a big house or buying new toys. The primary things are love and companionship. Divorce gives you another chance to make this discovery. If you do learn this, the rest of your life will be richer."

Along with the emotional ups and downs come physical changes. "Divorce is a major stressor, even when it's amicable, says Allan Rabinowitz, a Santa Monica stress-management expert. "If it's bitter, the impact can be that much worse. Tension soars, immunity may be weakened—possibly resulting in more colds and flus—and sleeping habits may change."

The period after a divorce may be the first time a man has lived on his own as an adult. His eating habits are almost sure to undergo a radical change, often leading to weight loss or gain. Studies show divorced men tend to drink and smoke more as well.

"Divorce is hard on your body," Rabinowitz concludes. "The antidote is to accept that this is a difficult time, that your symptoms are normal. And then take concrete steps, like focusing on health. Keep to an exercise program. Watch your diet in particular because a bad one can make dealing with the stress that much harder."

THE SEXUAL ANGLE

Minor sexual problems are so common after divorce that it's probably wise to expect them. A survey of 30 divorced men, published in *Sexuality Today*, showed that among men whose wives initiated the split—and in most cases it's the wife who does—impotence or premature ejaculation was common. During the first sexual encounter after the divorce, *all* the men had erectile problems, usually because they felt they were being judged by their new sex partner. The men who had initiated their divorces had fewer troubles.

"Many divorced men experience problems around dating and sex," says Bernie Zilbergeld, Ph.D., author of the book *Male Sexuality*. "A big reason is that as a marriage falls apart, so does the sex. His wife may have told him he's not a good lover, that she never had an orgasm, that he was too rough...too fast. He hears that he's basically an awkward sex partner, and he may carry this self-image with him into dating."

Here, too, there's a cure of sorts. "If you're not functioning sexually," Dr. Zilbergeld says, "that's a clue that you haven't emotionally finished with your ex-wife. This doesn't mean you have to talk it out with her. Usually you don't." Instead, he says, step back a few paces in the mourning process and get control over those postmarital feelings. Do it on your own, with friends or with a counselor. "Once you finish with her, you can get on with developing a new, effective self-image," Dr. Zilbergeld says.

A final postdivorce problem is limited to men with children, but for them it may be the toughest hurdle of all. In about 90 percent of divorces, the mother gets custody of the kids. "If you have children," says psychologist Diane Medved, Ph.D., author of *The Case against Divorce,* "a divorce will affect you emotionally for the rest of your life."

Rich Fowler (name changed), a Phoenix engineer, agrees: "I've been divorced 12 years and, whenever I see my daughter—she's 16 now—I remember the pain I went through." Carl Vaughan (name changed), a Washington, D.C., government employee, tells a similar story: "What I most regret about my divorce—really *all* that I regret—is that it cut me off from my son. He's 15. I haven't really known him since he was 5, and that hurts."

FASHION A NEW FATHERHOOD

Here, remedies are thornier. No matter how many bad feelings the divorce stirred up, staying on at least cordial terms with your ex-wife will help make the transition easier on the children. And it's usually not a good idea to be a "Disneyland Dad," unless that's the way you were before the divorce; kids usually just want to relate to their father the the way they always did. Beyond that, the best advice for divorced fathers is probably just hang loose and take each new situation as it comes. "If you're creative," Hartley says, "you'll find new relationships with your children."

Don't expect that new relationship to be inexpensive, however. Divorce can make the logistics of fathering extremely complicated. Take the case of Walt Dietrich (name changed), a Philadelphia-area executive whose 12-year-old daughter lives with him during the summer but with her mother in Minneapolis during the school year. Dietrich's effort to be a long-distance father from September through June involves numerous plane tickets, phone calls at 10 every weekday evening, faxing copies of report cards and the like...you get the picture. "It's worked well for the last three years," Dietrich says, although he realizes that soon he's going to be competing for her time at night and on weekends. "She's going to be on the phone with friends, hanging out on weekends with friends—like I did when I was a teenager," he says. "I'm already seeing a time when long distance won't be the next best thing to being there."

Given how divorce can thump a man's mind and body, not to mention those of the people around him, the rewards aren't always immediately evident. But to men who are going through a marital breakup and are having second thoughts, Mr. Rabinowitz offers some encouraging words: "You will survive. If you make the effort, you will recover. It may not be an easy process, but in the end, you'll have a more satisfying lifestyle." Divorce, he promises, "can be the key that unlocks a new, richer life."

—Robert McGarvey

Part 5

THE WOMEN IN
OUR LIVES

Flash! Men and Women
Are Different!

*Forget everything you've learned in Politically
Correct 101. There are at least 30 ways in which
men and women are different.*

• •

EVEN THOSE OF US who are politically correct enough to skip the pink-and-blue baby clothes have come to admit there are differences between the sexes that can't be ignored. Reality, it turns out, is heavily laced with yin and yang. From incidence of heart disease to tolerance of pain to strategies for seduction, men and women go their separate ways. Here are some facts and figures to prove it.

1. **Body talk.** The average adult U.S. male is 5-foot-9; the average female, 5-foot-4. He carries 1½ times as much muscle and bone as she does, and half as much fat.

2. **High hopes.** Men tack on an average of more than half an inch to their true height, while women subtract more than two pounds from their true weight, according to the Metropolitan Insurance Company.

3. **The longevity gap.** In the United States, women live 7.3 years, or 2,665 days, longer than men. At age 65, the ratio of surviving women to men is 100 to 65. Hang around. Gerontologist Steven Fox, D.O., says, "By following a healthy exercise regimen alone, men could increase their longevity by about 9 percent."

4. **Yeah, but what if *Sex* magazine had done the survey?** For men, money and sex are equally important, but for women, money is on their mind more often than sex, according to a survey by *Money* magazine. And more women said they *enjoy* money more than sex.

5. **Tab hunters.** More women than men take vitamins. An estimated 88 million women use vitamin and mineral products, compared with 81 million men.

6. **The burden of proof.** More than 8 percent of men are alcoholics, compared with only 3.5 percent of women, according to the National Institute on Alcohol Abuse and Alcoholism. Men can drink more than women before suffering health problems because their metabolism of alcohol is faster.

7. **"Not tonight, dear..."** Men suffer fewer aches and pains than women, reports *USA Today*. Women feel at least one symptom of discomfort (headache, fatigue, etc.) more than 43 percent of the time, compared with men's 28 percent. Then again, men find it twice as tough as women to take the same amount of chronic pain. Being in pain is also more likely to lower a man's self-esteem than a woman's.

8. **Remember the Maine vacation?** Women remember better than men, and the discrepancy increases with age.

In a word-recall test at Johns Hopkins Medical Institutions, men generally lagged slightly behind women; men in their late sixties scored a full 20 percent lower than did women of the same age.

9. **Eye-opener.** Men have a weaker sense of smell than women, but are more sensitive to light.

10. **Joint custody.** Males in their senior year of high school are only slightly more likely to have smoked marijuana (63 percent) than are women (56 percent), according to *Drugs in American Society* by Erich Goode. However, the boys were more than twice as likely to be daily users—10 percent versus 4 percent.

11. **No kidding.** We all can dish it out, but who can take it? According to *Psychology Today,* men and women equally resent criticism from their mates, but men take it more to heart when their kids put them down.

12. **Time's on our side.** The University of Iowa asked a group of managers how they would persuade a tardy employee to show up on time. More than 60 percent of the male managers but only 37 percent of the females said they would use warnings, criticisms and ultimatums. In contrast, 30 percent of the women but only 12 percent of the men said they would try a counseling approach ("Is there anything I can do to help you get to work on time?").

13. **Defense mechanism.** Men are more likely than women are to favor spending money on nuclear weapons, according to *Source* magazine. Men also tend to view military defense issues in simpler terms, while women tend to have a more complex perspective.

14. **Look who's talking.** Men converse mostly about news events and work; women talk mostly about food and health, according to a study published in *U.S. News and World Report.*

15. **Wheel difference.** Men drive more than twice as many miles as women annually: Men average 13,412 miles; women, 6,079.

16. **Can't touch this.** Women are more prone than men to get ripply fat—sometimes called cellulite—on their thighs

and buttocks because the fibers holding their skin to muscle are in parallel cords. This structure permits fat to bulge through and marble the skin. You seldom see cellulite on men because under the skin men have a dense mesh of fibers, which unites the fat in one smooth layer.

17. **Their loss is our gain.** A study of University of Michigan freshmen found that 85 percent of the women wished to lose weight; 45 percent of the men wanted to *gain* weight.

18. **Symphony for the devils.** To get a date, guys tend to boast about their past accomplishments and earning potential, and to show off their cars and stereos, according to a study in the *Journal of Personality and Social Psychology*. Women more often rely on their looks and may play hard to get or display sympathy for a guy's troubles.

19. **Provide and conquer.** Men tend to choose a mate based on good looks. For women, a man's looks are not as important as his social status and wealth, says David Buss, Ph.D., a psychologist at the University of Michigan.

20. **Close calls.** Men feel nearly as much need for intimacy as women but experience it differently, according to a study done at Loyola University of Chicago. For women, intimacy leads to more satisfaction in their roles as wife and mother. For men, being able to be close with people creates confidence and resiliency that lets them go out and conquer the world.

21. **Wild thing.** Men's preferred home activity is sex, while women's is spending time with the family (number two for men), according to surveys by R. H. Bruskin Market Research and Speigel.

22. **Doctored facts.** Men exercise more strenuously than women do, but they also smoke and drink more, finds a study at Pennsylvania State University. Women know more about nutrition, and they get more eye exams and dental and blood pressure checkups.

23. **Everyone out of the pool.** According to a Gallup survey, the most popular sport for men is fishing. Women's most popular sport? Swimming.

24. **The pits.** It may be indelicate to say so, but women's are smellier. Men perspire more heavily on their chests and women more heavily under their arms.

25. **Wake up, Irene.** Studies suggest that men spend more time in shallow sleep as they get older and may even start skipping deep sleep altogether, says Arthur Spielman, Ph.D., director of the Insomnia Treatment Center in New York. For unknown reasons, aging doesn't affect women's sleep as much.

26. **Left leanings.** Most men put their pants on left leg first, while the majority of women start with the right leg.

27. **Eat and run.** Men are 31 percent more likely to choose foods and beverages to improve athletic performance but find it more difficult to eat healthful snacks than women, according to a poll by HealthFocus, a Pennsylvania food consulting firm.

28. **A man's heart.** Men have double the risk of heart disease that women have, a tendency that some researchers attribute to the male hormone, testosterone. Evidently the hormone triggers the production of cholesterol. Men also have higher blood levels of stress hormones, which cause the heart to beat harder and blood pressure to rise.

29. **Bully for you.** A Norwegian study found that most school bullies are male, and that while the tendency of boys to bully rose with age, in girls it dropped. Researchers conclude aggression is partly biological in nature and, again, testosterone may be the spur.

30. **Dieting.** One out of three women diet, compared with one out of five men.

—Marc Bonanni and Susan A. Nastasee

• •

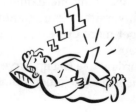

Do You Sleep in the Nude?
Twenty-six percent of American men sleep in the nude, up from 19 percent six years ago. The proportion of women who sleep bare is stuck at 6 percent.

Bridging the Gap

Just how wide is the chasm between men and women? This list may hold some surprises for you.

• •

OUR GOAL IN COMPILING the following list was never to dispute the existence of a gender gap. There's always been one, and always will be. Rather, we wanted to get a fix on just how wide that chasm is these days.

Pretty wide indeed, it turns out. For starters, with all the talk of equality, men are still society's leaders. The CEOs of 497 of the Fortune 500 companies are male. For their part, women continue to outlive men by an average of seven years.

Just what you expected? Perhaps. However, many of the statistics we uncovered defy conventional wisdom. For example, despite decades of "Just wait until your father gets home" stereotypes on television, it turns out that only 30 percent of men spank their children, while 71 percent of women do. And only 23 percent of women, but 35 percent of men, admit they've used a headache as an excuse to avoid sex. Read on for more surprises.

Average number of doctor's visits a man makes, per year: 4.5
Average number of doctor's visits a woman makes, per year: 6.2

Heaviest weight lifted overhead by a man: 560 pounds
Heaviest weight lifted overhead by a woman: 286 pounds

Fastest mile run by a man: 3:46.32
Fastest mile run by a woman: 4:15.61

Chance that a man will be struck by lightning: 1 in 1,800,000
Chance that a woman will be struck by lightning: 1 in 8,000,000

Chance that a man will become a high-ranking executive: 1 in 11
Chance that a woman will become a high-ranking executive: 1 in 20

Percentage of men who are college graduates: 22
Percentage of women who are college graduates: 16

Percentage of violent-crime victims who are men: 62
Percentage of violent-crime victims who are women: 38

Number of men on death row: 2,211
Number of women on death row: 33

Nobel prizes awarded to men: 588
Nobel prizes awarded to women: 24

Male members of American Mensa, the U.S. high-I.Q.
society: 35,139
Female members of American Mensa: 19,011

Chance that a man talks to himself: 1 in 12
Chance that a women talks to herself: 1 in 7

Percentage of men who would like to lose weight: 42
Percentage of women who would like to lose weight: 62

Percentage of men who like the way they look in the
nude: 68
Percentage of women who like the way they look in the
nude: 22

Percentage of men who snore: 53
Percentage of women who snore: 23

Chance that a man is color-blind: 1 in 25
Chance that a woman is color-blind: 1 in 50,000

Percentage of men who say they find a woman's face to be
her most attractive feature: 27
Percentage of women who say they find a man's face to be
his most attractive feature: 55

Chance that your best friend fantasizes about your wife:
1 in 2.5
Chance that your best friend's wife fantasizes about you:
1 in 6.6

Percentage of married men who have had an extramarital
affair: 37
Percentage of married women who have had an extramarital
affair: 29

Success rate, in a study, when men tested the pickup line "Hi" on women in a bar: 71 percent

Success rate when women tested the pickup line "Hi" on men: 100 percent

Percentage of men who enjoyed the first time they made love: 86

Percentage of women who enjoyed the first time they made love: 41

Average number of intercourse positions a man knows: 14

Average number of intercourse positions a woman knows: 9

Percentage of men who prefer sex with the lights on: 45

Percentage of women who prefer sex with the lights on: 17
—*Melissa Gotthardt*

Marriage of Opposites

As if all the other differences weren't enough! She's a morning person, and you don't really wake up till noon. Can this relationship be saved?

• •

IT'S 7:30 A.M. and my brain is a bazaar of voices: a radio weatherman, a dreamy woman's voice and a toddler insisting, "Wake up, Daddy!" Someone—the woman?—says gently, "Shhh, let your daddy sleep, Ben."

"I wanna vitamin, Mommy." And with this, I hear small footsteps padding away and a bittersweet voice saying, "It's Daddy who needs the vitamin," as I slip into a merciful half hour more of sleep.

At eight o'clock, I force myself to get up and make my groggy way downstairs. Two-and-a-half-year-old Ben bounds over and jumps on my lap. My wife, Debbie, even more of a morning person than Ben, has been up accomplishing things for hours already. The notion of early birds and worms crosses my mind. Good for birds, I concede, but for us worms, it's safer to sleep late.

After dropping Ben off at his day care, Debbie and I head to a nearby coffee shop, where I down three quick cups. Hours earlier, she had consumed a large and healthy breakfast, her big meal of the day. I find foodstuffs disgusting first thing in the morning.

"Thanks for letting me sleep late," I tell Debbie as the caffeine works its jangling magic on my nerves.

"I never mind it when you sleep," Debbie says. "Unless you're driving."

BODY CLOCKS OUT OF SYNC

She doesn't mind so that I won't mind when she sleeps. Debbie's energy peak for the day occurs at 10:00 or 11:00 A.M. By the late afternoon, just as I am really waking up and ready to plink away at my obligations, she is slowing down. I won't eat my dinner until 8 or later, a time when *she* finds foodstuffs disgusting. In fact, by then, she's already in her pajamas.

"Shhh," I find myself whispering to Ben as I wrestle him to bed around 8:30 P.M., "let your mommy sleep."

It's not until after midnight that I am at last ready to join Debbie for five overlapping hours in bed. She may be asleep, but her presence still comforts me. Call our relationship a generally successful "chrono-romance": two circadian mirror images who have managed to find more happiness than discord while living lives that are out of sync.

Relationships like ours, along with those of millions of other "dyssynchronous" American couples—perhaps as many as half of all couples—have attracted the attention of researchers who are fascinated by the impact of time on unions. Psychologists are looking at time from a variety of perspectives, not only the daily scheduling of sleep, work, sex and meals, but also the speed at which each partner moves and talks.

TIME IS THE ESSENCE

"Time is the very fabric of a relationship," says clinical psychologist Peter Fraenkel, Ph.D. "People living under the same roof but in different time zones, so to speak, may be more distressed than those that are geographically separated but on the same schedule. Time often goes unnoticed—or unacknowledged—as a source of conflict in a relationship."

Dr. Fraenkel recalls one couple who argued frequently about numerous problems, rarely coming up with any solutions. The root problem, Dr. Fraenkel realized soon after they came in for counseling, was not so much what they argued about but rather the different speed at which they argued. Sue, a 29-year-old corporate lawyer, usually initiated discussions and offered her opinion rapid-fire. Then she'd pause—briefly and impatiently—to let Ted, a 35-year-old wine-store owner, interject his remarks. If Sue's speech was set at 78 RPM, Ted's was stuck at 16. Because he tended to weigh his thoughts before sharing them, Sue often jumped back in before he could even start—leaving them both frustrated.

"A lot happens at that split-second interval in terms of who interrupts whom and how long pauses are between each person's turn," says Dr. Fraenkel. "People often get out of sync even at that level. And an awful lot of heartache that is attributed to other problems can stem from these rhythmic disturbances."

Once Dr. Fraenkel had pointed out the time dyssynchrony in their speaking styles, Ted and Sue were able to make conscious adjustments that led, in turn, to much more fulfilling talks. And each stopped imagining that the other's innate speech rhythms were intentionally designed to be irksome.

Getting a new perspective on time differences can be helpful. Early in my marriage, I would often try to cajole Debbie into discussing our finances late at night, when my energy and worries both peaked. She always became irritable, which I assumed meant that she wanted me to shoulder the money woes all by myself. I was convinced she was being selfish; she was convinced I was trying to wreck her night's sleep. When we eventually agreed to reschedule our financial talks earlier in the day, our money problems didn't magically improve, but our understanding of each other did.

HOUSECLEANING WOES

Another aspect of time that can create misdiagnosed conflicts in couples is the pace at which each partner tackles shared projects. Ralph, a 40-year-old security specialist, and Cindy, a 38-year-old administrative assistant, had been living together for over a year when they came to see Dr. Fraenkel for counseling. Their problem: They fought bitterly and frequently over household cleaning and maintenance chores. Cindy typically began early and worked without resting until the job was completed. Ralph, who was equally interested in seeing their house maintained, moved much slower; it took him longer to get started, and he liked to take breaks and pace himself as he worked.

Dr. Fraenkel advised the couple to view their respective rhythms not in terms of good and bad but as potentially complementary approaches. Over time, Cindy helped Ralph speed up a little and become more productive, and Ralph helped Cindy slow down and become less frantic.

Not all time problems have such straightforward solutions. As my wife and I have seen, when a morning person marries a night person, not only do they have less time to spend together but there is usually an accompanying *moral* dimension to their conflict. The morning spouse may brand his or her mate lazy for sleeping so late; the night spouse reciprocates by calling the other boring for never wanting to go out at night.

Jeffry H. Larson, Ph.D., assistant professor of counselor education at the University of Florida, Gainesville, decided to investigate the phenomenon scientifically. He and his colleagues studied 150 young couples from Utah, Montana and Alabama. After answering a set of questions, each spouse was classified as either a morning person, a night person or "undifferentiated." Further psychological testing confirmed much of what practicing therapists had already suspected: When a night owl marries a lark (a morning person), the couple fights more, socializes less, has sex less often and complains of loneliness more than a synchronous couple. Part of the problem is that a night owl/lark couple simply *has* less time together—up to 45 percent less, according to Dr. Larson's study.

IMPOSSIBLE SYNCHRONICITY

To make things worse, our internal clocks are tough to adjust, so it's sometimes impossible for such couples to force themselves into synchronicity. In a classic study, experimenters took the body temperatures of a group of volunteers every hour of the day for weeks. In morning people, body temperatures rose by one to two degrees before noon and then fell back to the baseline in the evening. Night people's temperatures didn't rise until 3:00 or 4:00 P.M. Energy peaks correlated closely to these physiological rises in temperature. "The biological research," says Dr. Larson, "suggests that our clocks are set early in childhood, and the most a person can comfortably change is an hour and a half in either direction."

But there's hope: The research also determined that mismatched couples (or at least those who worked out the inherent problems in their relationships) ended up with the best marriages of all. Such couples had better problem-solving and communication skills than even the happiest time-matched couples. Perhaps that's because they were forced to compromise and talk, a kind of marital sink-or-swim situation.

The study was not designed to determine how happily mismatched couples manage to cope so well. But therapists speculate that such couples adopt special strategies to minimize the impact of their dyssynchronies—for example, consciously planning everything from sex to conversations to socializing during hours when both partners have sufficient energy to enjoy them.

LEAN ON FRIENDS

Another strategy is to rely on social support outside the relationship: The lark meets morning friends for a sunrise jog, and the owl has night friends for a late movie. "The fact that I am a member of a dyssynchronous relationship," says one night owl named Clive, "has allowed me to go with my friends to see *Total Recall,* both *Evil Dead* movies and a host of films my wife wouldn't be caught dead at."

Beyond such specific tactics, however, successful chrono-romance seems to depend upon an almost philosophical approach to making things work that can be summed up in three words: accept, adapt and complement.

■ Accept that neither of you will ever be able to change your body clock. Don't try to convert her to your schedule or switch to hers. Instead, give in to each other's rhythms and look for common time—usually somewhere around the middle of the day—to enjoy each other.

■ Adapt the best qualities of your partner's work style to suit yours. If you're the type who thrives on fast-paced activity and chaos, and she approaches tasks methodically, you have a lot to learn from each other. If you appreciate each other for your differences, your relationship will be all the stronger.

■ Complement her weaknesses with your strengths (and vice versa). For example, the male half of one couple I know speaks of the greater reach that their out-of-sync schedules allow them. "Between the two of us," he says, "we really cover and utilize a lot of hours each day."

DISCOVER THE ADVANTAGES

It may be a hallmark of happily mismatched spouses that we search for ways to put a positive spin on our situations. We manage to discover advantages where less happy couples see only time incompatibilities. When Debbie and I drive long distances, for instance, we get sleepy at different times, making it easy to spell each other at the wheel. It may not be exactly true that our dyssynchrony has saved our lives on the highway, but what harm is there in thinking that it might have?

Another advantage I particularly appreciate is that each of us has some guilt-free time to read or just be quietly introspective without feeling we're slighting the other. But it's not only on a day-to-day level that our differences help us. I'm very future oriented and am always considering how best to help our family navigate a path in the years to come. Debbie is more reflective, our family's historian. She keeps track of where we have come from—and tempers my anxieties about the future with reminders of adversity overcome.

"To make things work," sums up Dr. Fraenkel, "you need to view dyssynchrony as rhythmic complexity. It's like when two drummers are playing—it's more interesting when they aren't playing the same thing. When two people's rhythms are different but intertwined, it forms a larger rhythm that is at once complex and exciting."

To those of us who have learned to dance to the music he's talking about, it's hard to imagine it any other way.

—*Jim Thornton*

• •

CLOCK WISE

Are you a night owl, a lark or something in between? Take our quiz and find out. After reading each of the following questions, circle the number that follows the response that best describes you. Add up the numbers to get your score and compare it to the scale at the end of the quiz.

1. If you were free to plan your day, when would you get up and when would you go to bed?

Get up (A.M.)

5:00 to 6:30	5
6:31 to 7:45	4
7:46 to 9:45	3
9:46 to 11:00	2
11:01 to noon	1

Go to bed (P.M.)

8:00 to 9:00	5
9:01 to 10:15	4
10:16 to 12:30	3
12:31 to 1:45	2
1:46 to 3:00	1

2. If you have to get up at a specific time, how dependent are you on the alarm clock to wake you?

Not at all dependent	4
Slightly dependent	3
Fairly dependent	2
Very dependent	1

3. How easy is getting up in the morning?

Not at all easy	1
Not very easy	2
Fairly easy	3
Very easy	4

(continued)

• •

• •

CLOCK WISE—CONTINUED

4. During the first half hour after waking up...
How alert are you?

Not at all	1
Slightly	2
Fairly	3
Very	4

How tired are you?

Very tired	1
Fairly tired	2
Fairly refreshed	3
Very refreshed	4

How's your appetite?

Very poor	1
Fairly poor	2
Fairly good	3
Very good	4

5. If you have no commitments the next day, when do you go to bed compared with your usual bedtime?

Seldom or never later	4
Less than 1 hour later	3
1 to 2 hours later	2
More than 2 hours later	1

6. Some friends want you to exercise hard with them. How would you perform...
From 7:00 to 8:00 A.M.?

Quite well	4
Reasonably well	3
Poorly	2
Very poorly	1

From 10:00 to 11:00 P.M.?

Quite well	1
Reasonably well	2
Poorly	3
Very poorly	4

• •

7. When in the evening are you tired and ready for bed?

8:00 to 9:00 P.M.	5
9:01 to 10:15 P.M.	4
10:16 P.M. to 12:45 A.M.	3
12:46 to 2:00 A.M.	2
2:01 to 3:00 A.M.	1

8. When would you be at your peak for:

A grueling two-hour quiz?

8:00 to 10:00 A.M.	6
11:00 A.M. to 1:00 P.M.	4
3:00 to 5:00 P.M.	2
7:00 to 9:00 P.M.	0

Two hours of exhausting physical work?

8:00 to 10:00 A.M.	4
11:00 A.M. to 1:00 P.M.	3
3:00 to 5:00 P.M.	2
7:00 to 9:00 P.M.	1

9. You've gone to bed several hours later than usual, but you can wake up when you wish to. What is most likely to happen?

You'll wake up at the usual time and stay awake	4
You'll wake up at the usual time and doze lightly	3
You'll wake up at the usual time but fall back asleep	2
You'll wake up later than usual	1

10. One morning you must be on watch from 4:00 to 6:00 A.M. You have no commitments the rest of the day. Which of the following would you do?

Would not go to bed until watch was over	1
Would take a nap before watch and sleep after	2
Would take a good sleep before watch and nap after	3
Would take all sleep before watch	4

Total Points

Score	
14–23	Night owl
24–31	Almost an owl
32–44	Neither (intermediate type)
45–52	Almost a lark
53–65	Lark (morning type)

• •

Don't Go Away Mad

The secret to getting along better with women may well lie in learning how to argue with them. Here are the rules every man should know.

● ●

WHY CAN'T MEN AND WOMEN GET ALONG BETTER? The prevailing view these days is that men are terrible at talking out their feelings. However, in studies of why couples split up, University of Denver psychologist and family therapist Howard Markman, Ph.D., found that hiding from emotions isn't the problem. "Men do just as well as women at communication and intimacy," he says.

The real issue, Dr. Markman discovered, is that we are so uneasy about arguing with the women we love that we often withdraw at the first sign of conflict. "Women mistake that for rejection, and often incorrectly believe that we don't want to express our feelings or aren't even capable of it," he says.

Many relationships collapse under the weight of all that miscommunication, in large part because couples aren't skilled enough at constructive arguing. But learning to argue better is a skill like any other. According to Dr. Markman, people can learn how to have better relationships. He and his colleagues have developed and tested a method he calls "Fighting for Your Marriage" to train people to better handle their disputes. We asked him to explain his methods and the thinking behind them.

Q. Why do men find arguing so distasteful?

A. First of all, we like to have rules for handling stress and conflict. In situations where men do really well—business, sports, war—disagreements are handled by following specific rules. It's something we're trained to do starting at an early age. Ever since preschool, for example, my son Mathew has loved kickball, a game which is guided by rules and relies on outside arbitrators such as adults or older kids to settle the inevitable disputes. In fact, even in warfare, there's a general convention for fighting. But there's no set of rules for couples to handle their disputes.

Second, a number of studies have shown that arguing actually feels physically different for men. It's more upsetting and unpleasant. Blood pressure, heart rate and all the other indications of how we respond to stress rise faster, higher and for a longer period in men. Without rules, men may feel more helpless in the face of a dispute and sometimes just don't know what to do.

Q. What happens in a typical fight?

A. It often starts with the woman bringing up an issue: "We have a problem with money" or "You don't talk to me" or "We need to spend more time together." Often, the man perceives what she's saying much more negatively than she's intending. Next, the guy—even if he's staying involved in the discussion—often signals in some way that he's not interested in talking. He withdraws, perhaps by turning away from her, rolling his eyes and saying to himself, "Here we go again." The woman then pursues the discussion, often in an increasingly negative way, and the man withdraws more. In our research labs, we make videotapes of couples doing this.

In many cases, the man may try to cut off the discussion by agreeing with her prematurely: "Yeah, you're right, so tell me what to do and I'll do it." This buries the issue and it will likely come back to haunt the couple later on. Or, sometimes, he may come back with something negative like "You're

• •

Which Buttons to Press to Drive Her Crazy

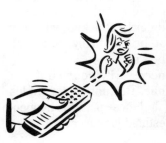

From a recent item in *Adweek,* news that should surprise nobody on the planet: Men are 14 percent more likely to take primary charge of television channel-changing, and it drives women berserk. In the interest of sexual harmony, you may want to relinquish your iron grip on the remote once in a while.

always attacking me. You're just like your mother," and all of a sudden they're really off into an increasingly negative cycle of attacks and counterattacks.

Q. It sounds as though men have good reason to think talking only leads to fights.

A. That's an interesting point because it may become a self-fulfilling prophesy. The more a man fears fighting, the more he withdraws and actually increases the chance of a fight occurring. The other part of the picture is that the woman usually misreads his withdrawal as something negative about her. This gets her angry or hurt—exactly what he's trying to avoid. Often the man then focuses on her anger, which in turn only upsets her more. Instead, he should focus on how he can avoid withdrawing. Watch out for blaming your partner. This is a danger sign. Both people actually feed the escalation process. The sad part is that they each start out wanting to do something positive.

Q. You've said that you can predict with 90 percent accuracy whether a marriage will succeed or not. What are the clues signaling that a relationship is at risk for problems?

A. There are three major danger signs. The first is that the man routinely withdraws from conversation.

The second is rapid escalation during arguments—for example, fights that erupt out of nowhere over embarrassingly trivial things. When disagreements don't get resolved, there's a buildup of negative emotions that explode like volcanoes. Some eruptions are predictable and some are not.

The third danger sign is invalidation. That's where, for example, the guy spends all Sunday cleaning up the house instead of watching football, and when his wife gets home she says, "You were going to clean the house, but the kitchen is still a mess." He feels he's been unfairly attacked, which is very damaging. If this happens a lot, he eventually starts feeling he's being attacked even when he's not.

Now, your relationship isn't necessarily doomed if you face these situations once in a while. But unhappy couples (and those at risk for unhappiness) find these patterns happening more frequently than couples destined for success.

Q. How can couples resolve their differences better?

A. One key is to establish certain ground rules for discussing issues in a way that isn't threatening. First you need to set up a regular time every week when both of you can bring up your concerns. Make sure you won't be interrupted—let the answering machine pick up calls while you're meeting, have the TV off and the kids asleep. The idea is that if you talk about issues in a structured, controlled way, they won't come up so often at other times, and when they do, you'll be able to discuss them more calmly.

Q. This sounds as if you're making an appointment to have a fight.

A. The way to keep that from happening is for both people to use what we call the speaker/listener technique, in which one person talks and the other just takes the words in. The speaker should keep the message brief and to the point, limiting comments to the issue at hand. Then, every few minutes, you reverse roles and the other person gets the floor.

Being the listener is the harder job. You need to make sure you're understanding what your partner is saying without defending yourself, agreeing or disagreeing. It's not a point/counterpoint debate but an attempt to see things from the other person's perspective. One important technique is to stop the speaker every 20 or 30 seconds and paraphrase what she's said to make sure that what you're hearing is what she means.

This method counters the three destructive patterns I mentioned earlier. It stops the man from withdrawing by keeping both partners active in the discussion, it confines escalation by allowing issues to be discussed in a controlled manner, and it prevents invalidation because one partner is continually affirming the other by paraphrasing. Any couple following this procedure should be able to have a constructive discussion about anything in their relationship. However, like any other skill, it takes practice.

Q. What are the potholes to look out for?

A. A lot of people prematurely try to solve disputes before both partners hear each other out. This is particularly true for men, who tend to want to fix problems, to "patch things up." Often, the issues don't actually need to be solved; 70 percent of the time, people just want to be heard.

Q. Are you suggesting we should avoid coming up with solutions for our problems?

A. The time and place for problem solving is after the issues are on the table. At first you may want to postpone talking about possible solutions until the next meeting. But as couples get better at this process, they can ultimately talk about an issue and solve it within 20 minutes or a half hour.

Q. What if you don't have anything you care to discuss?

A. You simply yield the floor. But there are ways of helping couples identify the ongoing issues in their relationships. We have simple forms people can fill out that are like a checklist of common areas of contention, such as money, sex, communication, kids, careers. There are always things to talk about.

If neither person really has anything to discuss, keep your appointment as a special time for just the two of you. Go for a walk, give each other back rubs, make love. It can be a lot of fun, although you shouldn't try to combine these talks with fun things. For example, don't go out for dinner to have your meeting. We find that when couples are doing something clearly defined as fun, they ban sensitive issues from their conversation. For a lot of couples, the best place to meet is the kitchen, over a cup of coffee.

Q. Is it possible to develop better relationship skills outside of the relationship?

A. It's generally easier to take what works well in an intimate setting and apply it outside the home than it is to take things that work well at the office, for example, and use them at home. A man is particularly likely to say, "Well, I'm good at this stuff at work, but not at home, so it must be her fault," which is not very successful thinking on his part. But it's not his fault, either. For example, on the job, men are highly reinforced for problem solving but not for listening. I often see airline pilots, lawyers, engineers and other professionals who are very successful in their careers, and may even see themselves as good communicators, but who become totally frustrated when they faithfully try applying what they do at work to their personal relationships. Also, we don't want our airline pilots to spend time talking about their feelings while they're landing a plane.

Q. What other guidelines do you suggest?

A. Establish a rule that either of the partners can bring up an issue at any time. You don't have to wait for the weekly meeting, and in fact you should try to deal with issues as soon as they arise. But the person who's listening has the right to say, "This isn't a good time." It's then the listener's responsibility to make sure that the issue gets discussed, preferably within 24 hours.

Q. What's the payoff of using these methods?

A. In our studies, we've seen divorce rates reduced by 50 percent and higher rates of marital happiness.

Because of AIDS and the growing perception that divorce isn't working as an option, people are now more motivated to have solid relationships with one partner. At the same time, it's harder for couples today because the roles for men and women are more equal than they were in the past. Suddenly, everything is negotiable, and there's a premium on problem-solving skills, which most people sorely lack.

You're in a relationship to have fun, to have a friend, to make love, maybe to have kids. You're not in it because you like conflict. But some conflict is inevitable. If you learn how to handle it, you'll be able to enjoy those other things to the fullest.

—Richard Laliberte

Talk That Talk

*Now that we've talked you into picking a fight
with her, you'd better learn how. A clue:
Speak the same language.*

••••••••••••••••••••••

IT WASN'T A FIGHT, it was a discussion. Well, remarks were exchanged. All right, maybe it was an argument. Okay, it was a fight—a 12-rounder. And after one particularly sarcastic retort on my part, my wife muttered, "You don't fight fair."

I was bewildered. What did she mean? I put together a pack of verbal fists and I smacked her with it. That's fair. This is a fight, lady. Unfair would be if I took out ads in the local papers listing her less favorable qualities. Then she might have cause for complaint. But mere sarcasm? Perfectly legitimate, in my book.

I have come to the conclusion that men and women simply fight differently and have conflicting ideas on what constitutes a fair fight. (In fact, men and women frequently disagree on what constitutes a fight. One person's knockdown, drag-out battle is another's calm, rational discussion. Basically, here are the points to remember: If you ended the exchange with a simple declarative sentence such as "I agree" or "That's true"or "I'll try to," that was a discussion. If you finish up with any of the following phrases: "Well, let's agree to disagree," "You know how much I hate that" or "Leave it where I threw it!" or if you use the name "Oprah" anywhere in a sentence, you were in a fight.

HITTING BELOW THE BELT

So how do men and women fight differently? Well, women have been known to pull some pretty rough stuff during an argument. For example, some women (who shall be nameless because she is sitting right next to me) have no hesitation in using tears. Using tears is not fair fighting because tears come naturally to many women but to very few men. We are frequently driven mad by women's tears and don't know how to respond, except by turning on the SportsChannel or reading Henry Miller, neither of which puts you in the mood for fair fighting.

Of course, I must admit that we men have some unfair techniques of our own. Here's one: We refuse to admit that a problem exists, then we follow it up with one of those long, cold, hurt silences that end only when the woman has either apologized or started to enjoy the quiet. The phrase that seems to enrage every woman in America, that has her seriously wondering just how far a single income can go, is that clenched-teeth male statement, "There's nothing wrong—I'm fine."

"Oh?" thinks the woman. "That must be why you're lying in a room with no lights on, curled up in a fetal position."

I must counter this, however, by pointing out that women have a habit of expecting you to know intuitively what's bothering them, a fighting technique that, if adopted by all the countries of the world, might destroy civilization as we know it—but would certainly save on the cost of translators at the United Nations.

We men like to argue, as long as it doesn't get personal. Women, you see, find that a contradiction in terms. When things get personal, we'll inevitably go for the jugular and say something that will be regretted by both parties for longer than a lifetime. (Shirley MacLaine still remembers several unkind things said to her one afternoon during the Paleolithic period.) We can tell she's been wounded: She gets that look in her eyes, the one that says, "I'm hurt more than I ever thought I could be. But I forgive you. You know not what you do."

At this point she has us where she wants us, and the only thing we can do is rend our garments and beg for forgiveness. And so the cutting remark, at first the male weapon, becomes hers.

ALL'S FAIR, EVEN NONSENSE

Women always reply to an offensive thrust with a defensive counterattack. Any minor criticism the man makes during an argument will inevitably be countered by her criticism of him. If he doesn't like where she puts the wall art, then three days ago his socks were out of place in the living room. It doesn't have to make sense; that's how it goes when fighting gets personal. For centuries, women were encouraged to define themselves by how the world saw them, and the effects still linger. Personal criticisms strike deeper in women than in men.

My wife (reading over my shoulder, which drives me crazy, and that's an argument we can have later) reminds me that women are totally bewildered by one aspect of men's fighting technique, the device which we call *feudus interruptus*. This refers to the astonishing ability we have to engage in verbal combat with all the venom of a rattlesnake, suspend the argument for a four-hour period while we are out with friends, be charming and outgoing with those friends as if nothing had happened, return home, walk through the front door and pick up the argument at the exact point where we left off, without missing a syllable. That woman you see standing in corners at parties talking to herself is not mentally unsound. She is merely trying to understand how her husband can be across the room linking arms with three friends and singing "Hey Jude" while she still has steam coming out of her ears.

But this is because men have been raised to believe that fighting is normal, commonplace and even healthy. Fighting is, I think, more disillusioning for women. Even today, a male in a relationship plays the role of the protector at least part of the time; more than that, in the best of marriages, the husband and wife are mutual best friends. Women see arguments as the world gone mad: Here is the protecting, trusting friend who suddenly turns on you, whipping off his Jimmy Stewart mask to reveal Freddy Krueger. Women feel genuinely betrayed by a fight; nothing is ever the same again. Men see an argument as, well, an argument. Continents haven't moved; mountains haven't crumbled.

NOTHING IS THE SAME AFTERWARD

In a sense, women are right. Nothing is ever the same again after a fight. But that doesn't mean things are worse. The relationship hasn't necessarily been terminally damaged. It may even be better. The world turns; it doesn't end. My wife and I think so. We've waded through these communication problems and emerged, if not unscathed, at least unbowed. We have come to understand some of the differences in what we each see as fair fighting and have arrived at some common ground. It's all in the art of compromise.

We've agreed, for example, to allow each other one low blow per fight—that is, she's allowed to criticize any one thing about me (but only something that I can change, like my mustache), and I'm allowed to say one thing that is so insensitive only a close friend or lover could think of it.

In addition, we've decided that fighting during meals or just before bedtime is out, since I can't concentrate on arguing when there's spaghetti being served anywhere in the continental United States, and she loses control over her short-term memory the moment she sees a comforter.

Moreover, we've achieved enough of a rapport to join forces in combating the alleged marital experts. For we've come to this conclusion: By-the-Book Fair Fighting is overrated. Yes, you should try to argue in an adult, moderate fashion, but in the how-to books, too much is asked of the couples involved. They are expected to have superhuman control of their emotions, egos and vocal cords. The last couple to fall into that category was Steve Lawrence and Eydie Gorme; unfortunately, most of us fight like Steve Martin and Idi Amin ("Well, excuse me!" and "I'll have you cold for breakfast").

So we've consulted with friends in the same situation and come up with our own, extremely flexible, suit-your-own-needs kind of rules, what we call "The McDonoughs' New and Improved Rules for Fairly Good Fighting." For example:

The experts say: Avoid conflict by using an open-ended question ("What would you like to do tonight?"), using multiple choice ("Would you like to go out or stay home?"). If you follow this line, you will not appear manipulative.

We say: You will also not appear alive because your mate will have throttled you by now for asking the world's most incredibly maddening series of questions.

The experts say: Disregard negative statements. A hurt or angry mate is likely to couch the problem in exaggerated, accusatory terms.

We say: It's pretty hard to disregard the expression "You toad-sucking primordial swamp ooze." And why should you ignore the hurt? Don't you have the right to acknowledge the pain caused by what the other person has said? What are you, a neutral bystander?

The experts say: Stick to the issue. Don't bring up something that happened two days ago.

We say: Just don't bring up something that happened in a previous generation. It's okay to say, "And you watched *It's a Wonderful Life* seven consecutive times last year, and you only let me watch *Mr. Magoo's Christmas Carol* once." It is not all right to say, "And your Aunt Edwina, in 1921, put a flower in her hair and danced down Broadway in the nude." Not only is this not fair fighting, but it necessitates calling somebody's mother to get out the photo album and see if the incident was documented. This takes up the whole evening, and there goes the chance to finish the fight.

The experts say: Don't end by saying something that will never be forgotten.

We say: I've spent my whole life trying to think of something that will never be forgotten. If it comes to me, do you really think I'm going to let the opportunity go by? I can always apologize to my wife later, but how often do I get a chance to score in *Bartlett's Familiar Quotations?* Which brings us to the last rule.

The experts say: Don't go to bed mad.

• •

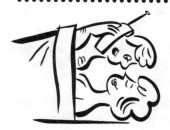

If a Man Answers
If the phone rings during inter-course, 60 percent of men and 65 percent of women let it ring. Of those who answer, 12 percent of men and 20 percent of women stay busy while on the phone.

We say: What if you're already in bed? Should you get up? In the final analysis, it is important to fight fair and to find ways to fight that are acceptable to both people. But couples are incapable of fighting like the emotionless automatons in the how-to books, and if they set their expectations too high, if they believe that fighting is always a sign of trouble, they will be constantly disappointed. A certain amount of disagreement in a relationship is inevitable. In addition, no two people, male or female, fight exactly alike. Ultimately, you have to let your love and respect for each other take over the argument and hope for the best. There are no instant and easy solutions. And probably there aren't supposed to be. Just wear adequate rain gear for the weeping sessions, bring a good book for your wife to read while you are indulging in one of your silences, and realize that the words "I'm sorry" never hurt and frequently help. And then you can make up. But that's another story.

—*David McDonough*

Part 6

SEX

Up from Impotence

*When you're hot, you're hot. When you're not,
there's plenty of help available. A noted urologist
explains the options.*

....

WAITING FOR THE FRONT DOOR to buzz me into the Park
Avenue office of New York City urologist E. Douglas
Whitehead, M.D., I get the feeling the doorman next door is
scoping me out, thinking "Geez, that guy couldn't be more
than 34, 35 maybe. Awfully young to be having trouble getting
it up."

I want to explain that I'm just a writer who's come to do a story. There's nothing the matter with *my* equipment. Luckily, I'm saved from making a complete fool of myself by the release of the electric lock.

Minutes later I'm in a warm, comfortable office filled with framed color prints, where one of the founders of the Association for Male Sexual Dysfunction has put me at ease talking about a subject that makes a lot of men, even a lot of doctors, uptight.

Soon hydraulic penile implants cover his desk like so many Datsun spare parts. He pumps each model up to its maximum hardness and at one point holds a plastic vacuum pump to the crotch of his slacks and demonstrates it by pumping the device.

Maybe he's not as uninhibited as the British urologist who capped a lecture at a national meeting of the American Urological Association on drug treatments for impotence by pulling down his pants to show off his drug-induced erection ("About eight years ago and we're still talking about it," Dr. Whitehead says), but clearly he's no shrinking violet on the subject of sexual medicine.

Were all urologists as down-to-earth and up-to-date as Dr. Whitehead, the world would be a much happier place for the 15 to 20 million American men who suffer from impotence. Unfortunately, only about a third of urologists in the United States make impotence and male sexual problems a significant part of their practice.

Dr. Whitehead considers the situation very unfortunate: "At worst, physicians can reflect the same embarrassment that the public often feels in talking about impotence," he says. "Too frequently, I hear about doctors who will slap a patient on the back and say, 'Be realistic. You're over 60, you've had enough sex. Just accept it.' But I see patients in their seventies and eighties who are beginning to have trouble getting an erection and *very much* want to do something about it."

If doctors don't talk about impotence, many men won't get help, which is sad because, according to Dr. Whitehead, 90 percent of cases are treatable, usually without surgery. We asked him to elaborate on the latest developments.

Q. What's new in impotence treatment?

A. The big news of the last ten years is we've discovered that emotional and psychological problems do not cause most cases of impotence. Advances in mapping the blood flow in the penis have shown us that approximately 75 percent of impotence is organic (physically caused).

Q. How can you determine if impotence is actually a psychological problem or a physical one?

A. We interview the patient, using an eight-page questionnaire as a guide. A man usually does not have a physical problem if, for example, he can get an erection during masturbation or during sleep, or if he fails to get erections with one sexual partner but succeeds with another. After the interview, we perform a physical examination, including examining the genitals and looking for signs of excessive female hormones. We also test the pulses to the lower extremities and do a regional neurological exam.

Then, if the problem appears to be psychological, we usually refer the patient to a sex therapist or to a psychiatrist.

Q. What's the most common physical cause of impotence?

A. The most common one is arteriosclerotic plaque forming on the walls of the penile arteries—a possible consequence of high cholesterol levels in the blood. This narrows the diameter of the vessels that carry blood to the penis. When your body can't deliver enough blood to engorge the penis, it doesn't matter how turned on you are. You will not be able to get or maintain an erection. Sometimes we see other vascular problems, nerve disorders or hormonal problems, but they're rare.

Q. What kinds of options does a man have?

A. For physical impotence, the available treatments include penile implants, penile injections, vacuum-constriction devices, hormone therapy and occasionally other forms of surgery. Medicare and other medical insurance policies generally cover treatment costs for organic impotence.

Q. Let's discuss these treatments one at a time. How do penile implants work?

A. There are two general types: noninflatable and inflatable. To understand how they work, you need to picture the anatomy of the penis: It has two channels within the shaft, one on the left side and one on the right. When not enough blood supplies these channels or when too much blood drains out, they cannot fill and expand and become rigid. So penile prostheses are implanted, one in each channel, to take over the job of the blood in making the penis erect.

The noninflatable types use a semirigid or bendable rod in each channel, giving you an erection. The rods can be bent by hand. You bend them down close to the body to conceal your penis while dressed; you bend them up into an erection angle to have intercourse. The disadvantage is, there is always a solid shape in the penis that you can feel, and the penis doesn't expand in width like it does with the inflatables.

The inflatable implants use two hydraulic cylinders that can be pumped up with fluid. One model is self-contained, with the fluid reservoir and pump combined in the cylinder itself, so the whole system is implanted in the penis. You pump the front tip of the penis several times to inflate an erection. You bend another site downward to drain the penis.

The second kind of inflatable model uses a separate fluid reservoir hidden in the belly and a pump hidden in the scrotum. And the latest models incorporate the reservoir and the pump together in the scrotum. When you're ready to have sex, you feel for the bulb under the skin of the scrotum and press it several times, inflating the cylinders in your penis with fluid. The erection will stay hard for as long as you want, even after ejaculation.

Q. How satisfied are patients with implants?

A. Both types have a success rate of over 90 percent in terms of satisfaction of the patient and his sexual partner. That's the highest success rate of any of the treatments. Another measure of their success is that when there is a malfunction, almost everybody wants the device replaced, not just removed. That, to me, shows they were happy with it.

Q. In the last two devices you mentioned, how natural-seeming is the erection? Would a woman notice anything odd?

A. It appears so natural, a sexual partner might not be able to tell the difference; it can be that good cosmetically. There is only a little scar concealed by the pubic hair, or a little scar on the front of the scrotum, depending on the model and the surgeon's choice of incision.

Q. Is there discomfort for the man with any of these devices?

A. After a week or two or three, most men don't have any discomfort. They say it becomes like part of their body; they don't even think about it being there.

Men with implants can have orgasms and ejaculate, and if they are fertile they can even father children.

Q. The most recent development for impotence is penile injections. How do injections work?

A. There are three types of medication that we use in various combinations and doses: papaverine, phentolamine and prostaglandin-E_1. They all cause the blood vessels to dilate, engorging the penis with blood.

The patient can ask the doctor to determine a dose for an erection that lasts for a half hour, an hour, or an hour and a half, whatever he chooses. But certainly not more than four hours. And with the injections, you should not have sex more than eight or ten times a month.

Q. A needle in the penis doesn't sound like it would exactly put you in the mood for sex.

A. The drug is injected at the base of the penis with a very short needle that has a tiny diameter. The patient feels a little pinch, if that. The erection usually comes on in 5 to 15 minutes.

Q. What about vacuum devices?

A. You place a suction tube over your penis to draw blood into it, then a constriction ring is slipped off the base of the device onto your penis, trapping the blood inside. After sex you slip off the constriction ring and the erection becomes soft.

Q. What are the disadvantages?

A. For some men the stability is not so good. The ring only hardens the outer two-thirds of the penis, the visible part. So it's a wobbly erection, but usually hard enough for penetration.

••

HELP WANTED?

Where to call for information on impotence.

Impotents Anonymous, 2020 Pennsylvania Avenue NW, Suite 292, Washington, DC 20006. Send a self-addressed, stamped envelope for free information; phone (301) 731-1988 for information about patient support groups around the country.

Impotence Hotline, (800) 558-4321. For general information, pamphlets and physician listings, write to Surgiteck, 3037 Mount Pleasant Street, Racine, WI 53404.

Impotence Information Center, P.O. Box 9, Minneapolis, MN 55440; (800) 843-4315. Write for the free booklet "Impotence Help in the USA," or call toll free.

The phone directory. Dr. Whitehead suggests looking up urologists and selecting one who specifically advertises treatment of sexual impotence, or calling the urology department of a local hospital or medical school for a referral.

••

There can also be a little discomfort, a tightness of the skin, but most patients get used to it. The success rate is 70 to 80 percent, but a lot of men don't want to bother with a vacuum device because it seems so unnatural and cumbersome during foreplay. In my practice, very few patients choose it.

Q. What about hormone therapy?

A. Hormonal problems occur in less than 5 percent of cases. Of those, the most common problem is that the testicles don't produce enough testosterone, the male sex hormone. Occasionally, a problem with another hormone, prolactin, is discovered. I refer all such patients to an endocrinologist. The testosterone-deficient patients receive hormone injections once a month. The outcome is usually successful. The patients with a problem with their prolactin can usually be successfully treated with a medicine called bromocriptine.

Q. Sounds like there are good solutions, yet studies show that more than 60 percent of impotent men put off going to a doctor for at least a year. Many wait five or ten years. What would you say to someone who's begun experiencing problems?

A. There's absolutely no reason to keep impotence a secret any more than, say, diabetes. The medical profession has to help this process along. Impotence and its treatment is just now starting to be taught at medical schools. And urologists in particular need to help make their patients more comfortable. They too are making strides, now that effective treatments are available. I think slowly the taboo is being lifted.

—Mark Canter

Where Did Our Love Go?

Sex may very well turn out to be the prime casualty of the 1990s. Do we have to wait until the next millennium to get back our lost love?

• •

WELCOME TO THE 1990S, the Era of Almost Sex. We watch it, read about it, talk about it, joke about it, worry about it, argue about it, use it to sell tires and vodka, go to museums to see pictures of it and pass laws against it.

Everything but *do it.*

"The yuppies sure aren't doing it as much," says Ted McIlvenna, Ph.D., of the Institute for Advanced Study of Human Sexuality in San Francisco. "Sex frequency hadn't changed since the 1950s, but there's been a decline in the past few years. I don't think the decline is because of AIDS. I think it's because of stress. Sex is no longer a priority, and that's scary."

It certainly is for Patrick Allen (name changed), a 33-year-old health professional in northern California, married for 12 years to a social worker. "My wife and I invest so much time and energy in our careers that usually we don't have anything left for sex," he says. "The stresses in my life build up. There's always something: patients' demands, my own demands on myself, personnel hassles, billing problems. Sometimes I get

• •

DON'T HURRY, BE HAPPY

The pressures of a high-achieving career have resulted in more young career men seeking treatment for premature ejaculation, says Sheldon O. Burman, M.D., director of the Male Sexual Dysfunction Institute in Chicago.

"Men who become premature ejaculators are often responding to an unhealthy lifestyle, particularly stress on the job or in a personal relationship," says Dr. Burman. "Those at high risk include men who don't handle stress well, can't relax, have too much work and constantly feel hurried."

Other factors that can play hell with your sex life include excessive smoking or consumption of alcohol or drugs. Even being on a poor diet or being overweight can cause premature ejaculation and other forms of impotence, which affect more than 20 million American men.

Premature ejaculation can be particularly straining on a relationship. "Women bear a special hardship in cases of premature ejaculation because they are often hurt the most by the problem," says Dr. Burman. "Frequently, when a man regularly ejaculates prematurely, he shuns all forms of intimacy and communication. The woman feels rejected and wonders whether she has become unattractive to him. She begins feeling guilty, thinking she has done something to upset him. And then she becomes suspicious, wondering if he has a girlfriend somewhere."

If the problem isn't psychological, treatment for premature ejaculation usually consists of learning how to handle stress or making other lifestyle changes—including things you'd never think to associate with sex, such as quitting smoking and improving your diet.

• •

home and I just feel depleted—emotionally and sexually. When I first realized this was happening, I tried to make love anyway, but that didn't work. I began having erection problems."

For many men, it seems, life in the fast lane has meant passing right by sex. One study of happily married couples found that when it came to sex, 50 percent of the men reported a lack of interest or an inability to relax. A sex life that's been stalled by the time pressures of two-career relationships is one of the most common reasons couples seek therapy, says psychologist Peter A. Wish, Ph.D., director of the New England Institute of Family Relations. "Some call it the yuppie sex problem, but it affects couples of all ages and incomes. Sex becomes an afterthought. These couples work hard, come home beat, make dinner, put the kids to bed and collapse in front of the TV until bedtime. They'd like to make love but just can't seem to find the energy."

And as if lack of time weren't enough of an obstacle to a satisfying love life, many men are also suffering from "low sexual desire," which is often a physical symptom of chronic stress.

THE LOST URGE

"To tell you the truth, I just don't seem to need it much anymore," says Mark Shoner (name changed), 40, a West Coast financial analyst. "I never thought I'd find myself saying this, especially not at my age, but the urge doesn't strike all that often these days."

Shoner lives a very stressful life, full of bumper-to-bumper commutes, deadlines, disappointments and abrasive personalities. Although he doesn't fully understand why, he intuitively knows that the constant tension in his life is linked to his diminished sex drive.

"My girlfriend and I vacationed in Hawaii for nine days last year, and by the third day I was feeling like a young stud again," says Shoner. "We spent the better part of two afternoons making love.

"Then I went back to work and the tide ebbed away again, if you know what I mean."

We do. And we know why. Stress and sex are mismatched bed partners. In fact, by one estimate, stress is the culprit behind as many as 80 percent of erection problems. "People are not surprised when they're under stress and their stomach is upset, but they don't realize that erections can be affected by the same things," says Richard E. Berger, M.D., a Seattle urologist and coauthor of *BioPotency: A Guide to Sexual Success.*

STRESS STRIKES

Among the physical effects of stress is an excess of adrenaline in the blood. This "fight-or-flight" hormone directs blood to flow into muscles while at the same time constricting vessels in the penis. The extra blood needed to produce an erection can't get in. Daily stress can leave your system with an excess of adrenaline that's still there hours after work.

Stress can also reduce the level of testosterone, the male sex hormone responsible for sex drive. One study of soldiers in Vietnam showed that their testosterone levels dipped as they prepared to go to the front for combat and increased again when they returned from battle.

"Testosterone is an on/off kind of hormone," says Joseph LoPiccolo, Ph.D., psychology chairman at the University of Missouri in Columbia. "You only need a little to turn the sex drive on. But stress can depress the level to the point where sex drive turns off." Alcohol, which many men use as nonprescription medication for stress, can also reduce their supply of testosterone.

How we interact with others when we're under stress can

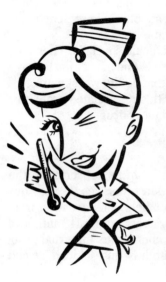

Naughty Nurses Tell All

Straight from the blazing pages of the *Journal of Sex & Marital Therapy,* here are the results of a sex survey of 709 professional female nurses. Those who generally experienced orgasm after their partners tended to be less sexually satisfied than those who usually reached orgasm before their partners or simultaneously with them. When the women were asked what changes they'd like to see in their sex lives, the most frequently mentioned desires were: more foreplay, more frequent intercourse, more romance prior to intercourse, more orgasms and more tenderness by partner.

• •

SEX AND DRUGS—EXPERIENCING TECHNICAL DIFFICULTIES

"A few years ago, one of my assistants gave me a lapel pin that said 'High on Stress.' It was perfect," says a 40-year-old Los Angeles television producer we'll call Barry Hoff. "I've always led a high-stress life: business breakfasts, impossible shooting schedules, obnoxious agents, union headaches. If anything, the excitement turned me on."

One day, while he was at his health club, Barry noticed a coin-operated blood-pressure machine. He popped in a quarter and learned that his was dangerously high. The next day, his doctor prescribed Inderal, a common blood pressure medication.

Not long afterward, following a particularly stressful week in which a big film deal fell through, Barry failed to get an erection while making love to his girlfriend. "Nothing like that had ever happened to me before. My girlfriend blamed herself. I blamed myself. Neither of us knew what to think."

Stuck in freeway traffic a few days later, Barry punched his way up and down the radio dial. "I wound up listening to a talk show with a sex expert who said blood pressure drugs can destroy erections. The guy named my drug, Inderal. I got on the car phone and called my doctor. 'Oh, yeah,' he said, 'Inderal can do that.' I thought, So why did you put me on it? He switched me to something else, and my erections came back."

According to San Diego sexual-medicine specialist Theresa Crenshaw, M.D., "Prescription drug use is one of the most overlooked factors in sex problems; drugs that do the worst damage are the medications men use to deal with stress-related problems: antihypertensives, antidepressants and ulcer drugs.

• •

contribute to sexual difficulties. A lot of us subscribe to the male ethic that we shouldn't burden other people with our problems and complaints or ask for help when we're in trouble. Oakland sex therapist Bernie Zilbergeld, Ph.D., author of *Male Sexuality,* says this behavior contributes to sexual problems indirectly by "making men withdraw and act irritable and

••

"I've seen many cases where a man under stress gets depressed or develops high blood pressure, and his doctor prescribes medication without mentioning that it might cause sexual side effects. Then the man loses his erections, and he gets even more depressed or his blood pressure goes higher."

Among blood pressure medicines, says Dr. Crenshaw, "the beta blockers cause terrible problems. Inderal is absolutely one of the worst." Other sex offenders include Aldomet, Aldoril and clonidine.

Less sexually debilitating alternatives, according to E. Don Nelson, Pharm.D., associate professor of clinical pharmacology at the University of Cincinnati College of Medicine, are the diuretics Capozide, Diuril and Dyazide; the ACE inhibitors Prinivil and Zestril; and the calcium channel blockers Adalat, Cardizem and Procardia.

Until recently, every commonly prescribed antidepressant could cause libido and erection problems. Dr. Crenshaw says, however, that Wellbutrin, a newer drug, "causes no sex problems. In fact, it may increase libido for some patients."

Throughout the 1980s, the ulcer drug Tagamet was one of the nation's most frequently prescribed medications. Unfortunately, it can put out too many fires, says Dr. Crenshaw. "A newer drug, Zantac, is equally effective but has fewer sexual side effects."

Alcohol is probably the nation's leading sex-stopper, she adds. "It's a central nervous system depressant. Drink enough and you simply cannot raise an erection."

••

weird. That turns women off. Women like to relate. They draw sexual energy from the communication and togetherness of the relationship. When men under stress pull away, women often suffer a loss of libido as well." Meanwhile, of course, the emotional withdrawal itself makes the man less likely to initiate sex.

SEX AS PREVENTION AND CURE

Ironically, sex is one of nature's best stress *relievers*. "Sex is healthy," says LoPiccolo. "It helps us sleep better and feel less stressed."

So how do you snap out of the downward spiral of stress, loss of sex drive, more stress? Making sex a higher priority can make it less of a chore. Dr. Wish recommends that couples who can't find the time to make love go on "sex dates. Go away for the weekend. Spend some quality time together."

These days, Patrick Allen and his wife make a point of taking a long, leisurely weekend every few months. "Recently we drove to a bed-and-breakfast inn about three hours away," he says. "On the way up, we caught up on each other's lives. When we got there we immediately went to bed—to take naps. We woke up refreshed and ready for sex. Afterward, we went to dinner and a movie. I never force myself to have sex anymore. When I feel a loss of sexual energy, I take it as a sign that I need to make more time for myself and for my marriage."

Don't feel you always have to have intercourse to have sex, especially if you're so stressed that the best you can muster is a ten-minute quickie that's about as exciting as washing the car. Some sex therapists recommend calling a moratorium on intercourse while you and your partner learn to become intimate with each other again. It can actually be quite a turn-on to plan a no-orgasm-allowed sex date. You can make out, massage each other—in fact, do anything but bring each other off. It takes the focus away from the genitals and orgasm as a proving ground.

RELAX AND ENJOY

For couples who are having severe sex problems, Dr. Berger often prescribes a six-week ban on intercourse. For the first three weeks, they're to schedule half-hour lovemaking sessions, five times a week, in which they refrain from touching either genitals or breasts. "The idea is to relax and enjoy the pleasure of being close without any expectation that intercourse will take place," he writes.

In the following three weeks, genital and breast touching is permitted but intercourse is still avoided. After that, the couple may enjoy intercourse—and often, even men with erection problems are ready to go at this point. If not, they return to caressing—or consult a professional therapist for direction.

Many men who are fully functional but whose desire has ebbed find that a regular exercise program miraculously jump starts their sex drive. Being in shape makes you feel better about yourself, more relaxed and arousable—more alive.

"Exercise can release hormones that counteract stress damage and provide feelings of mastery and well-being," says New York City psychologist Allen Elkin, Ph.D., a certified sex therapist and corporate stress consultant. "Even modest physical activity helps. Take a walk at lunch. Use the stairs instead of the elevator. Park a little farther from the front door of the office."

As for all the stress gadgets marketed in those glossy catalogs, Dr. Elkin says, "Men love machines, so biofeedback monitors and galvanic skin response meters can be useful in the early stages of stress-management training. But once they can recognize their own calmness, most men outgrow the machinery."

Remember, sex is not one of life's challenges. It's supposed to be fun. Of course, fun can be elusive—you know when you're having it, but if you try too hard, you won't. Still, it seems pretty clear that if, instead of stress, you bring to bed with you a willingness to play, your body will respond instinctively. Sex is one of the few areas where we adults are *allowed* to play. Take advantage of it.

—*Michael Castleman*

Intimate Moments

Men have such a hard time really talking
about sex. But it is possible to take sex talk
out of the locker room.

••••••••••••••••••••

ANY MAN WHO'S EVER PONDERED the difference between
the sexes is bound to settle on one crucial point: women enjoy
talking; men don't. We see it all the time—the women in our
lives are capable of happily spending an hour talking to a
friend on the phone, while we could be out in a fishing boat
with a buddy for a whole day and hardly compose a complete
sentence.

When the topic is sex, the communication gap between
men and women is particularly wide. Early on, women learn to
express their feelings, to talk about their fears and problems;
men, on the other hand, are taught *not* to speak of personal
matters.

But women's verbal fluency, especially in sexual matters,
can make men uneasy.

"Guys view intimacy as a one-to-one thing with their partner," says Alan S., 30, a lifelong bachelor from Chicago.
"Women, unfortunately, view it more as an open topic of discussion with their friends."

"I don't understand why women *have* to tell one another
what they did in bed with you the night before," says Isaac G.,
19, a college student from upstate New York. "I just don't
get it."

To Alan and Isaac and others like them, the sexual openness of women often seems like a betrayal. But some would
argue there's a flip side—that by being tight-lipped with each
other, we men are actually missing out on something good.
We may not be familiar with all the nuances of lovemaking
technique or the full variety of women's desires, but we'll be
damned if we're going to ask. "We're more likely to talk about
how to strip a car than how to strip a woman," says Bill L., 33, a
construction manager from Atlanta.

Men lost in a strange town will drive around aimlessly for hours rather than ask for directions. It's the same thing with sex. Many of us feel that to admit we don't know something is to reveal a serious weakness.

TALK IS THREATENING

"I think the point is that if men talk about their sex lives, it could put them in an embarrassing or threatening situation," Bill L. adds. "Women are talkers and sharers; men are not."

If men could get beyond their natural defenses and talk openly about their sexual experiences, as women often do, what would they say? In interviews with a number of men between the ages 18 and 42, *Men's Health* posed the question simply: "What *don't* you talk about when you talk about sex? And why not?" The answers were honest and enlightening, even if they required some effort to extract.

One of the touchiest subjects that came up was "performance problems." Experts say occasional bouts of impotence are extremely common among men. However, if it happens to a man once and he doesn't talk to anyone about it, doesn't find out how common it is, he may develop a fear that it's a permanent problem. And that fear can make it one. "Men often have fears of performance that they don't talk about," says Sheldon

• •

Just a Simple Hot Dog Will Do

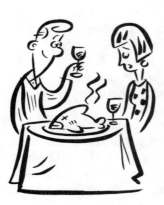

A tip for first dates: Don't take her to that new Vietnamese restaurant with the super-spicy food. A study by two Clemson University researchers found that men tend to have a stronger preference for hot, spicy foods than women do. You might want to skip the Japanese place that's famous for its blowfish sushi, too, since the study found that men are also more likely than women to seek out new and unusual foods.

Burman, M.D., a *Men's Health* advisor and founder of the Male Sexual Dysfunction Institute in Chicago. "And so they can become terrified during sex."

Rob D., a married office manager from Virginia, remembers a bad experience from his college days. He'd met an attractive 19-year-old woman in a bar where he was working nights and he took her home. They quickly tumbled into bed, but he was unable to get an erection. If she had been more understanding of his plight, everything might have turned out okay, but, perhaps because of her age, she perceived his problem as an insult. She was furious. The experience still haunts him. "I wish I had that one to do over," he says.

How much better things turned out for Tom R., a 33-year-old ad copywriter, when he decided to talk with his partner about a temporary bout of impotence. He was on vacation in Napa Valley with his new 27-year-old girlfriend. "We were away for two weeks, having sex two, three, five times a day. After the third time on the third day, I couldn't get it up."

LEARN TO COME CLEAN

"When I woke up the next morning, I said, 'I'm sorry about last night...I guess it was just too much.' Then she said, 'Are you kidding? I'm glad you brought it up. I thought it was my fault.'"

With the rediscovered emphasis on monogamy and marriage, we made it a point to ask early on whether men ever worry about sex with one partner getting boring.

"No, I'm not really worried about that," says Tom O., now in his fourth year of marriage. "The whole idea of conquest just isn't that important anymore. And frankly, I had a real active sex life before I got married. I stored it up; it was fun. I can remember it. There wasn't anything I wanted to do that I didn't do...twice. The sampling chapter of my life is behind me."

Tom sounds too mature, almost smug, as he says this. But then he tells us to call him back the next day, when his wife won't be around. When we do, he admits that, with some past girlfriends, sex sometimes became routine. As for his wife, he says, "if necessary, we'll keep sex interesting and special by having it less often."

Tom says any need to see other women has disappeared from his life, even before his first child was born last year. He acknowledges, though, that his mind has a little healthy lust still kicking around. "It's a vice, like anything else. And you'll always be battling what's left of it."

GUILT IS A BIGGIE

Guilt seems to be a big factor preventing married men from becoming entangled with other women. But that obstacle can fall away if the circumstances are right.

Rob D. didn't think about his one affair as much as he simply acted it out. "I'd been flirting with this woman I worked with for a year and a half," he said. "We'd go out to dinner every once in a while after work, no big deal. I'd even gone to her parents' house for dinner once with my wife. We were all friends. But when our company went out of business, the last day the whole office went out to lunch and got drunk.

"Two bars later, she asked me to walk her home. I did, and that's when she told me she'd wanted to have sex with me for a long time. And so we did. It was okay, but not great. We were both pretty drunk."

Great or not, the one-nighter remains a fond memory for Rob. He'd do it again if the conditions were favorable, which is to say without any planning or sneaking around.

Although few men will freely admit insecurity about their bodies, many, when prodded, will acknowledge it.

"A couple of years ago I was making out with a woman on my couch," recalls Vince P., 36. "It was getting really heavy when she whispered, 'I'm not wearing any panties.' God, I was hot, but when she asked whether she should spend the night, I told her I didn't think it was a good idea."

FEAR OF FAILURE

After some initial evasion, Vince admits that, at the time, he was nearly 20 pounds overweight and would have felt uncomfortable being naked in front of a stranger, particularly since he'd had problems in the past with impotence. He didn't want to risk a poor debut.

A few other men expressed similar fears. Craig M., a former high school wrestler, says he's sometimes embarrassed by his weight when he's in bed with his wife. "There are times when I wish I were more fit. Because I've been in the kind of shape where I've had less than 4 percent body fat. Nowadays, I feel like I used to in the off-season. You know, like a slob."

Brian N., a lawyer, remembers that when he was in high school and college, his short stature ("five four and *a half*") caused him to doubt his sex appeal. But soon after college, he began to feel more comfortable with his height. "I realized that some women are afraid of big, huge guys and so my being short made them feel less threatened.

"I'm short and I'm handsome," Brian says. "And I'm a kind man. Women appreciate that."

Dr. Alfred Kinsey, the great-grandfather of the modern sex researcher, reported back in 1948 that male masturbation is nearly universal. But not all men realize that,. and there's a great deal of guilt associated with masturbation, particularly among married men.

"Once I asked my wife, 'Don't you ever do it?'" says Vince P. "She said, 'Not very often' and looked at me as if it's something I should be ashamed of. So that was the last time I mentioned it. And, naturally, I don't do it in front of her, even though I used to in front of my old girlfriend. I'm sure she thinks instead of masturbating I should be saving myself for her."

SILENCE IS THE REAL SELF-ABUSE

Should men be able to talk more freely about masturbation? (After all, entire how-to books are written on the subject for women.) Rob D. is skeptical: "If you already know how to do it, what's there to talk about?

"I think it's nothing more than a momentary spontaneous release," he continues. "Men just do it because it feels good and it's entertaining."

Still, because the subject is so rarely discussed, misconceptions abound. Ron H., 35, an advertising copywriter, tells how as his wedding day approached, a younger colleague mentioned, "Well, I guess you'll never have to [masturbate] again."

"For a minute I didn't know what he was talking about," recalls Ron. "Then I realized that to his 22-year-old mind, getting married meant giving up masturbation forever. Well, I can tell you that it sure didn't in my case."

• •

STUCK IN LOW GEAR

Few couples are a perfect sexual match. More often than not, one partner would prefer sex more often than the other. Compromises are made and the relationship goes on.

In some cases, however, one of the partners has little or no interest in having sex at all. Doctors call it inhibited sexual desire (ISD), and it's a potentially serious problem.

ISD is not the same as impotence. The equipment still works, but the desire isn't there to fuel it. The sufferer is rarely in the mood for sex and may have difficulty becoming aroused on those rare occasions when sex takes place.

If you or your partner has a chronically flagging libido, the critical first step toward turning things around is to get the problem out in the open and talk about it. Don't make accusations or assess blame; just discuss it.

Sometimes the roots of ISD are medical, so the sufferer should see a doctor. Tests can rule out possible causes such as illness, severe stress, hormonal deficiencies, reactions to medication or depression.

If physical problems are ruled out, suspect an unresolved conflict in the relationship. It could be that performance anxiety, fear of intimacy or rejection, bottled up resentment or lack of trust has built an invisible wall down the middle of the mattress. If you and your mate are very open, very smart or very lucky, you may be able to resolve these conflicts by yourselves, but seeing a professional therapist will markedly increase the odds of success.

The good news is that ISD can usually be cured once the underlying causes are dealt with.

• •

It used to be said that men cared very little about pleasing their partners in bed, the old "Slam, bam, thank you, ma'am" thing. Then, as part of the sexual revolution, women began to speak up about their wants and needs. Our impression is that men have reacted to those requests. In fact, some of the men we spoke to seem more concerned with their partners' pleasure than their own.

FOREPLAY'S THE THING

Bob M., 37, a divorced marketing consultant in the San Diego area, takes no chances: "To me, foreplay is an art. I can go two, three hours at a time. I get as much enjoyment out of foreplay as I do out of intercourse."

Jack R., 35, a restaurant manager in New York City, considers himself "very sensitive" to a woman's needs, but he admits that he wasn't always that way. "When you're 23, you just want to get 'in there.' I don't remember the women I was with ever having orgasms. Maybe they did, but I wasn't focused on them or their pleasure as much as I am now."

What caused the change? Jack tells of his relationship with an experienced partner who showed him what turned her on, introducing him to the subtleties of touch and sensitivity that he was oblivious to when he was younger.

You don't have to be a genius to see that this kind of openness—with one's wife or girlfriend—is important to a healthy, lasting relationship. As for blabbing to your buddies about the minutiae of your sex life, that may be going too far. Most experts we talk to are in favor of staying in the framework of what's comfortable for you. If it doesn't feel right, they say, it probably isn't.

The truth is, we men have our own ways of communicating. Sometimes without uttering a single word. As Alan S. puts it: "One guy asks another how it went with some woman last night; he smiles and shakes his head slowly from side to side. And that's the entire discussion. But it speaks volumes. I can use my imagination, and those few gestures mean a whole lot more than any blow-by-blow description."

—Curtis Pesmen

The Sex Effect

*Is it a good idea to score before the big game? Let's
settle this question once and for all.*

● ●

THE MOST ATHLETIC DAY of my life was also one of the
most sexual. I was 25 and clinically depressed. To bludgeon
my mood into submission, I was exercising two to three hours
each day and attempting to have sex as often as possible.
Admittedly, this latter strategy proved difficult since it wasn't
all that easy to meet women who were attracted to a lugubri-
ous, unemployed guy with a tendency to weep.

On this one wonderful occasion, however, I *did* meet such
a woman—or, should I say, the recent divorcée met me. After
we'd danced together until 2:00 A.M., she whispered that she
felt "like a cat in heat." My mood lightened as I intuited my
role in her psychodrama. We went to her house and had sex
five times, a personal record for me.

The following morning I awoke early, sapped but san-
guine. I was scheduled to play a best-of-five-games racquetball
match against a court nemesis I'd never been able to beat.
The match lasted over two hours, and I won. Later that afternoon, my masters swimming team had intramural time trials,
and to my utter astonishment, I swam my best times since
college.

How could such breakthrough athletic accomplishments
be *possible,* I found myself wondering. Had I not, only hours
before, had sex to the point of virtual dehydration? Had not
every coach in every sport I'd played since puberty warned,
albeit obliquely, that sex before competition makes for a limp
athletic performance? My high school swim coach had even
gone so far as to advise us "to avoid impure thoughts during
the swimming season."

COACH WAS WRONG

Avoid impure thoughts? My life now was nothing short of
one long, uninterrupted impure thought and (mercifully) a lit-

tle action, too. And still, I'd successfully pushed the envelope of my athletic potential.

Was my experience just some kind of sampling error, or could it be that my coach was a knucklehead? (His only other consistent item of precompetition advice, I should point out, was this: "For quick energy, eat a box of dry Jell-O a half hour before you swim.") If my coach was wrong, he was certainly not alone. The "sex wrecks you" hypothesis appears in the literature of cultures as diverse as the ancient Hindus, Chinese folklorists and Victorian physicians. In such views, not just the body but also the mind can be spent by sex. Writer Gustave Flaubert, a usually perceptive chronicler of the human condition, reportedly exclaimed after ejaculating, "There goes another novel!"

In the United States in the late 1930s, a researcher named J. Dollard brought a certain scientific validity to such notions when a paper of his entitled "Frustration and Aggression" was published by the Yale University Press. The gist of the so-called Dollard paradigm was that abstinence leads to frustra-

Cure for Blue Balls: Lift a Truck

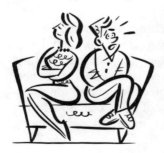

You can cure testicular ache brought on by prolonged, unrelieved sexual arousal by diverting the blood flow elsewhere, says Ray McIntyre, M.D., in *Medical Aspects of Human Sexuality*. He recommends straining against an immovable object—but not, presumably, the woman you were making out with. Rather, try lifting a car bumper for three or four seconds. That usually does the trick within the next 30 seconds. If it doesn't, you may need to repeat the exercise. (To save your back, be careful to squat and lift with your legs.)

tion, which leads to aggression, which leads to more vigor on the playing field. Dollard provided little empirical data to support his theory, but it didn't seem to matter since his notions resonated so harmoniously with what coaches and athletes alike already "knew" was the case.

To this day, soccer fans in Peru blame their country's loss to Poland in the 1982 World Cup on several players who indulged in sex the night before the game. Even some athletes who eschew pregame celibacy still believe sex affects them. One professional baseball pitcher, for instance, claims sex *does* drain him, but it's a *good* draining, which leaves him "a little tired" the day after, so his sinker ball drops more.

SCIENCE SPEAKS

Of all athletes, football players and boxers remain the most smitten with Dollardism, despite increasing evidence that the theory really doesn't hold up under much scrutiny. Consider the Minnesota Vikings: Before each of their last four Super Bowls, they separated their players from their wives. They lost all four games.

"Muhammad Ali told us that when you don't get sex for a while, you get mean and angry, and it makes you a great warrior," says Gabe Mirkin, M.D., an associate professor at Georgetown University's school of medicine. Dr. Mirkin pauses before adding: "It's a myth."

Since Dollard, studies of the impact of sex on trained athletes have been remarkably few. In a 1968 article published in the *Journal of Sex Research,* researcher Warren Johnson compared the grip strength of 14 married male former athletes, average age 28, on the morning after sex, and then after six days of abstinence. Johnson's conclusion: Strength and endurance of the palmar flexing muscles are apparently not adversely affected early on the day following nocturnal coitus.

Other than Nintendo, of course, it's hard to imagine too many sports where success hangs on the palmar flexing muscles. In an attempt to survey a broader range of athletic parameters, researchers at Colorado State University repeated Johnson's protocol on ten fit, married men ranging in age from 18 to 45. This time, however, the scientists measured not only grip strength but also balance, lateral movement, reaction time, aerobic power, maximal oxygen consumption and perceived exertion. Loren Cordain, Ph.D., a professor in the school's Department of Exercise and Sports Science, says that the as-yet-unpublished study found no significant difference in any of these measures following either sex or five days' abstinence.

"I'm going out on a limb as a scientist," he says, "but we have no reason to believe that any physiological parameter we can measure that's associated with sex is likely to be altered by sexual intercourse."

FURTHER...UH...STUDIES NEEDED

Until further studies can be done with a larger sample group that includes elite athletes, Dr. Cordain concedes that definitive proof of the "sex *doesn't* wreck you" hypothesis will remain elusive. Until then, diehards like my ex–swim coach are likely to keep on citing anecdotal proof—such as the Peruvian World Cup postcoital soccer loss—of the old thinking. But for every antisex anecdote, there are stories that suggest Dr. Cordain and Johnson are right.

Consider this: In the 1972 Olympics in Munich, the just-married middle distance runner, Dave Wottle, reportedly was still honeymooning the night before the 800 meters. Unfazed the next day, Wottle ended his race with a ferocious kick and won the gold medal.

Dr. Mirkin says he's heard of a boxer who won a fight shortly after masturbating in the elevator at Madison Square Garden. (Apparently nobody asked *why* he did this, or if he took off his gloves first.) Another athlete set a world record in a sprint following a similar precompetition "warm-up." There is even a legend circulating at the New York Road Runners Club about a male marathoner who had sex *in the middle* of a competition. He was running with his girlfriend, who decided to quit halfway through the race. He accompanied her to a motel, had sex, then went back and finished the marathon.

"I have worked with a large number of athletes," says Bob Arnot, M.D., medical correspondent for CBS News and Editorial Advisor to *Men's Health*. "Most of them—even the night before they compete in Olympic Games—can safely have sex without any real detriment to their performance. I

• •

CAN MAKING LOVE MAKE YOU FIT?

So sex is okay before exercise. How about sex *as* exercise, we wondered. On average, sexual intercourse burns up about 100 calories per hour, according to calculations done at the University of Rome. (Out of politeness we didn't ask *how* they were done.) Clothes-tearing, position-inventing, furniture-breaking sex can smoke up to 250 calories per hour. Compare that to running (880 calories per hour), tennis (536) or even *weeding* (330). Ejaculation itself is more demanding at 400 calories per hour, but since the longest ejaculation on record lasted about 15 seconds, you can only count on losing about 1 calorie there.

Your heart rate can escalate to 180 beats per minute during lovemaking. But this rise is not caused by the muscles' increased demand for blood and oxygen as it is in sports; rather, it's a hormonal reaction triggered by the exhilaration of sex. When you make love, your heart doesn't *work harder;* it only *beats faster* (and the speedup causes little increase in circulation). You get a similar boost in heart rate in response to fear—not to mention from drinking a cup of coffee. "You can't get a training effect, or get fit, from making love," concludes Gabe Mirkin, M.D.

• •

know people who have gone on to win bronze, silver and even gold medals the following day."

If anything, Dr. Arnot says, he recommends having sex the night before, especially for those athletes who are having trouble calming down enough to get a good night's sleep. "Properly timed," he says, "I think there's a tremendous benefit to sex before an athletic event. There is probably no better natural antianxiety drug available."

It's been 13 years since my serendipitous encounter with that divorcée. I'm married now, no longer depressed and still hoping to set a personal record in the 100-yard freestyle. In a couple of months, the annual state masters meet is coming up, and I'm determined to be ready. All that remains is to work out hard, and then buy a box of Jell-O. It's not for the meet—it's to give me the energy I'll need on the night before.

—*Jim Thornton*

Part 7

DISEASE-FREE LIVING

The Wonder Drug in Your Medicine Cabinet

*Take a look at aspirin's newly discovered benefits.
You may be in for a few pleasant surprises.*

••••••••••••••••••••••••

PERHAPS IT'S TIME to stop thinking of aspirin as that 100-tablets-for-$1.99 pain reliever you take when you have a mild headache. Although it's been a medicine-cabinet staple for more than 100 years, researchers have been taking a new look at it, and some of their conclusions are startling. In fact, when you look at all the therapeutic claims made lately for aspirin, you might wonder what ills it won't prevent—sometimes even with small doses.

Men's Health sent its research staff out to explore the latest aspirin studies. The researchers turned up the following list of the drug's newly discovered benefits.

REDUCES RISK OF HEART ATTACK

Aspirin's role in preventing heart attacks is probably its strongest credential. There now seems to be little question that an aspirin tablet every other day can help prevent that first heart attack and can be helpful to those who have had one already.

How does it work? First, we know that aspirin's main biological effect is to limit the production of substances called prostaglandins. And we know that one of the duties of prostaglandins is to promote blood clotting. So regular doses of aspirin help keep blood from clumping together, which reduces the likelihood that an artery will plug up and cause a heart attack.

In the Physicians' Health Study, a long-term study of over 22,000 healthy male doctors, those who took a standard 325-milligram aspirin tablet every other day had 44 percent fewer heart attacks than those who didn't. The researchers were so impressed by the results, they stopped the trial in midcourse and put all the doctors on aspirin.

REDUCES RISK OF STROKE

While nearly all research has shown that aspirin reduces the risk of heart disease, its effect on stroke is much more controversial. Of ten major studies conducted between 1977 and 1988, six have shown a reduction in stroke risk for those taking aspirin, while four have shown no effect. So the results are less than conclusive.

When those studies are divided into categories, however, some patterns emerge. First, aspirin has been shown in most trials to reduce the chance of recurrence in those who've already had a stroke. And second, it seems to help those who have other circulatory problems, such as irregular heart rhythm, chest pains and heart disease. In one study, patients with a rhythm problem called atrial fibrillation had 50 to 80 percent fewer strokes when given aspirin.

REDUCES RISK OF COLON CANCER

An American team reported in the *Journal of the National Cancer Institute* that when they compared 1,326 colorectal cancer patients with 4,891 cancer-free patients, those without tumors were much more likely to be regular aspirin users. In fact, the aspirin users turned out to have one-half the risk of developing this disease.

REDUCES RISK OF CATARACTS

The risk of getting cataracts is related to blood glucose levels, and there's some evidence that aspirin reduces the rate at which the body uses glucose. So British researchers tried administering aspirin and the aspirin-like medication ibuprofen to 300 patients. They found that the users of all three drugs were half as likely to develop cataracts.

BOOSTS THE IMMUNE SYSTEM

Aspirin has been found to increase the production of three important immune system chemicals: interleukin-2, interferon-gamma and interferon-alpha.

While researching this effect, scientists also tested aspirin's potential for warding off a cold. Although the subjects enjoyed no added protection from that common ailment, they did produce less mucus when they caught a cold.

PROTECTS AGAINST GALLSTONES

Scientists in the United States and Britain decided to see how aspirin would affect people with known gallstone risk factors such as high-calcium or reduced-calorie diets. Reporting in *Lancet* on 75 of the at-risk people they surveyed, the British researchers found that the 12 regular aspirin users developed no gallstones, while 20 of the 63 nonusers did. In the *New England Journal of Medicine,* U.S. scientists reported that of 68 adults on weight-loss diets, aspirin users developed fewer gallstones than those given a placebo.

REDUCES FREQUENCY
OF MIGRAINE HEADACHES

Aspirin is not a remedy for a full-blown migraine attack, but taking it on a regular basis seems to reduce the *frequency* of the attacks. In the Physician's Health Study, doctors taking aspirin every other day reported 20 percent fewer migraine attacks than those who got placebos. This finding is supported by a similar British study that showed regular doses of aspirin led to a 29 percent reduction in migraines.

RELIEVES HAY FEVER SYMPTOMS

According to a report in the *Annals of Allergy,* aspirin is as effective as some antihistamines in treating pollen allergies. One 41-year-old allergy sufferer enjoyed relief from symptoms for up to eight hours after taking aspirin.

MAY BECOME A FLU CURE

According to a letter in the *New England Journal of Medicine,* aspirin in very high doses can completely halt the activity of influenza virus. The dosage required is far too high to be given orally to humans, but researchers speculate that an aerosol form sprayed into the nose might someday be effective in controlling flu in the respiratory system.

Aspirin is so inexpensive and readily available that it's easy to forget it really is a drug. In fact, it's so potent, many researchers think that if aspirin were discovered or invented today, the Food and Drug Administration would restrict its availability to prescriptions. The main reason you can buy it freely is that it's been around so long.

Aspirin is not without its side effects when used in large doses. It can slow blood clotting, produce ulcers and cause tinnitus, an annoying ringing in the ears.

It would be wise to talk to your doctor before beginning a regular course of aspirin. Even if he says okay, don't overdo it. The optimum dose for cardiac benefits seems to be one regular strength (350-milligram) tablet every other day. When you take it in higher doses or more frequently, not only do the side effects increase, but some of the benefits may disappear as well (see "Why Not Once a Day?" on page 158).

• •

WHY NOT ONCE A DAY?

In a British study of over 5,000 doctors, a daily dose of aspirin did not significantly protect the doctors from heart attack, but an aspirin *every other day* did. Yes, it would be a lot simpler to take an aspirin every day—or even half an aspirin. Unfortunately, that simply doesn't work.

One explanation has to do with the specific prostaglandins that aspirin affects. For example, aspirin suppresses thromboxane, a blood thickener. Unfortunately, it also suppresses prostacyclin, a prostaglandin that inhibits blood clot formation.

It seems that when you take a dose every other day, blood-thinning prostacyclin has time to return to normal, while blood-thickening thromboxane stays suppressed, producing a net gain in blood-thinning potential.

Another reason to stick to an every-other-day dose has to do with immune system enhancement. When researchers gave their subjects aspirin every day, their immune systems were boosted at first but then ebbed back to normal levels. When the people got aspirin on alternate days, however, immune levels remained at a much higher level.

• •

That said, taking aspirin may well be the cheapest, most effective preventive there is—other than regular exercise and eating less fat—for a variety of illnesses.

—*Dave Schoonmaker*

Bet against Cancer

Cancer is not inevitable. These dos and don'ts from America's top 200 cancer experts could lower your risk considerably.

••••••••••••••••••••••

IF YOU READ THE NEWSPAPERS enough, you might get the impression that just about everything on the planet causes cancer. Hardly a week goes by when there isn't some new front-page scare. In the past few years, everything from apples to water has been implicated as a potential cause of cancer.

This barrage of dire warnings may at times leave you feeling a bit glum. If even fresh fruit and tap water cause cancer, there must be no way to avoid it. And if it's going to get you anyway, why think about it?

Men's Health felt that a little perspective was needed. Cancer strikes only about one in three people. Clearly, for most of us it's neither inevitable nor unavoidable. But because many of the cancer hazards talked about in the media are significantly less worrisome than others, it's become increasingly difficult to get our anticancer priorities straight.

For example, which is more important, checking the radon level in your basement or eating a high-fiber breakfast cereal? Losing weight or avoiding food additives? Going for cancer screenings every year or keeping a positive mental attitude? Knowing these things, it would be possible to develop a rational anticancer plan for yourself.

We felt that the right place to go to get that perspective was to the doctors and scientists on the front lines of cancer research and treatment. We asked Medical Consensus Surveys, a research arm of Rodale Press, to poll 200 experts at the 44 National Cancer Institutes–designated cancer centers in the United States. These physicians and researchers treat large numbers of patients, conduct full-scale tests of new cancer treatments and have access to the most up-to-date information available anywhere.

• , • • • • • • • • • •

THE TOP 15 ANTICANCER MEASURES

Here's how our experts rated specific actions that can help lower your cancer risk. One action, "Avoid industrial/agricultural toxins," scored high enough to be in fifth place, but it is not included in the top 15. These substances are associated with cancer risks, but exposure to them is confined to workers in certain industries rather than the general population.

Rank	Action
1	Don't smoke or chew tobacco
2	Get regular cancer screening tests
3	Perform testicular self-exams
4	Limit exposure to sunlight
5	Avoid high alcohol intake
6	Avoid "passive smoking"
7	Reduce overall dietary fat
8	Eat more food fiber
9	Eat more fruits and vegetables
10	Eat more whole-grain, high-fiber cereals
11	Maintain normal weight
12	Avoid household toxins
13	Get regular exercise
14	Limit exposure to nitrites
15	Eat more cruciferous vegetables

• •

We asked these specialists to prioritize risk-reducing actions by checking one of five categories: Extremely Important, Very Important, Important, Not Important (But May Help) or Probably Worthless. Their responses were analyzed to reveal a priority list of actions you can take right now to lower your risk of cancer (see The Top 15 Anticancer Measures above).

One extremely significant point that emerged from the survey: Half of our experts agreed that 50 to 70 percent of all cancers could be prevented if everybody followed the top-priority changes in lifestyle and diet outlined below.

KICK THE NICOTINE HABIT

As we expected, tobacco use leads the list of risks: Nearly all of our 200 experts say it's extremely important to avoid smoking or chewing tobacco. "If all the smokers in this country quit tomorrow, 30 percent of all cancer deaths could be prevented," says Edward Trapido, Sc.D., an epidemiologist at the University of Miami School of Medicine.

That's not just deaths from lung cancer, either. Smoking causes cancers of the mouth, larynx and esophagus, as well as body parts that don't have direct contact with smoke, notably the pancreas and the bladder.

Tobacco has been a highly publicized risk for nearly 30 years, but the warnings have all been aimed at the smoker. Within the last 10 years, passive smoking—exposure to tobacco smoke from others—has surfaced as a major concern. Over half of our respondents feel that avoiding passive smoking is either very or extremely important.

"The latest information I've read says that a nonsmoker's cancer risk increases 50 percent if he lives with a smoker," says William Shingleton, M.D., retired director of the cancer center at Duke University Medical School. Working eight hours a day in a smoky environment can also raise your risk.

CUT DOWN ON ALCOHOL

Nearly half the doctors rated avoiding high alcohol intake as very or extremely important. Alcohol in moderation seems to be a negligible risk. But the heavier drinker—14 or more drinks a week—has a greatly increased risk of cancers of the mouth, throat and liver. That's bad enough on its own, but it's a double whammy to the heavy drinker who also smokes, an all-too-common combination.

AVOID TOO MUCH SUN

Essentially all of the more than 500,000 cases of non-melanoma skin cancer each year are caused by too much sun, says Paul F. Engstrom, M.D., of the Fox Chase Cancer Center in Philadelphia. "The good news is that nonmelanomas are highly treatable, so considerably fewer cancer deaths are attributable to sun exposure."

The bad news: Recent evidence links excessive sun exposure to those rarer-but-deadly melanomas. That's part of the reason more than two-thirds of our respondents consider sunlight a very to extremely important risk factor.

GET SCREENED

Regular cancer-screening tests and self-exams are methods of early detection rather than cancer prevention. We included them in the survey because early detection leads to a better chance of a cure—preventing death rather than the cancer itself. Our respondents agreed. Getting regular checkups and doing self-exams garnered second and third places (after quitting smoking) on the "Top 15" list of cancer-preventing priorities on page 160.

The most important do-it-yourself tests for men are testicular self-exams. (After a warm bath or shower, gently roll each testicle between your thumb and fingers, feeling for any hard lumps or irregularities.) Testicular cancer is the leading form among young men, and if detected early, it's better than 90 percent curable. It's also smart to keep an eye out for suspected skin cancers. And for men over 40, one of the most important physician-performed screenings is the colorectal cancer test. You can also get screening tests for prostate, skin, thyroid, mouth and lymph cancers.

KEEP WEIGHT DOWN AND EXERCISE UP

As recently as ten years ago, doctors would have dismissed being overweight as a cancer factor. But since then, studies have linked obesity (defined by the American Cancer Society as being 40 percent or more overweight) with increased risk of colon, prostate and gallbladder cancers.

Exercise is crucial in controlling obesity, and our experts rate regular exercise to be of only slightly less importance than maintaining normal weight. It's difficult to establish a direct link between exercise and cancer prevention, but some evidence exists, for example, that people with desk jobs and sedentary lives are at higher risk of colorectal cancer. "Exercise may help reduce that risk," says Peter Greenwald, M.D., of the National Cancer Institute headquarters in Bethesda, Maryland.

THINK POSITIVELY

The notion that mind and body are interrelated is just coming into acceptance by the medical community. Among the doctors in our survey, 54 percent rated having a positive mental attitude as important, very important or extremely important. Only 22 percent labeled it probably worthless. A few years ago, those percentages would easily have been reversed. Recent studies show that stress-reducing techniques can cause measurable changes in the immune system. Whether or not these changes can help prevent cancer is still speculative. "It's hard to prove scientifically that a positive outlook can help prevent cancer. But many people—doctors, too—have a feeling that people with a positive attitude may smoke less and have better eating habits," says Dr. Greenwald.

• •

Sofa Spuds
of the World...Get Up!

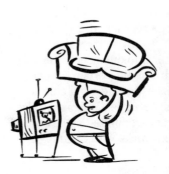

A sedentary lifestyle is the top risk factor for heart disease, greater than high blood pressure, obesity, diabetes, smoking or high cholesterol, reports the Centers for Disease Control (CDC). Inactivity (less than 20 minutes of exercise three times a week) was nearly twice as deadly as the next killer, high cholesterol. But if sofa spuds began to take daily brisk walks for 30 minutes, says a CDC expert, the added activity could save more than 22,000 lives each year *in New York State alone.*

CONSIDER YOUR ENVIRONMENT

Environmental factors scored surprisingly low in importance on our survey. While they are still considered risks, most of our experts think that most are not serious causes of concern.

Electromagnetic fields. About a third of our experts think it's ridiculous to worry about electromagnetic fields from high-tension wires, electric blankets, computer screens and so on. In fact, the magnetic-field category was the second-lowest risk on the entire list. "It's a very, very, very rare cause of cancer compared to smoking and sun exposure. But people tend to overestimate the risk of outside factors they can't control," Dr. Engstrom explains.

Radon. This one is a little more controversial. The Environmental Protection Agency (EPA) maintains that radon is the second most important cause of lung cancer, right after smoking. The EPA's warning is based primarily on studies of miners exposed to radon miles underground. Can we accurately relate those findings to the risk aboveground?

"I don't believe there's a shred of epidemiological data to relate household radon exposure to cancer—nothing that links cancer clusters and high-radon areas," states J. John Cohen, M.D., Ph.D., of the University of Colorado Medical School. Yet probably because the American Cancer Society backs radon as a potential risk factor, 47 percent of our doctors still say it's important to check the radon level in your home. The rest seem to be on the fence: Over 26 percent say it isn't important but it may help. Very few of the experts picked the extreme responses.

Toxins. Industrial and agricultural toxins scored high as risk factors. There is solid research linking certain industrial agents (such as nickel, chromate, asbestos and vinyl chloride) to increased cancer risks in workers. Farm pesticides may also pose hazards to farmers. But the risks are limited since only a relatively small part of the population works with carcinogenic chemicals on a daily basis.

Twenty years ago, you'd be hard-pressed to find a doctor who'd say that diet had anything to do with preventing cancer. Things have changed dramatically, and our survey shows it.

Most of our experts rated dietary habits important, very important or extremely important.

"Dietary factors probably account for up to 35 percent of all cancers. That's according to a landmark National Cancer Institute–sponsored report," Dr. Trapido states. And this figure is higher than the figure for smoking. (Not a big surprise, since everybody eats and only a minority still smoke.)

Chemicals in your food. There are a number of items in our survey that can be termed "dietary chemical hazards." Like the environmental risk factors above, these chemicals have reputations that are far worse than their scores on this survey.

Nitrites, which are used to cure bacon, hot dogs and other meats, received the most concern from our experts. Nitrites have indeed been associated with increased cancer risks.

Washing fruits and vegetables to remove chemical residues may be a good health practice, but it counts as only a moderate risk-reducer. Concern with food additives scored toward the bottom of the list in importance. As with other chemicals, frequency of exposure is the key to determining risk. Eating fresh fruits and vegetables and avoiding high-fat prepared foods limits contact with preservatives.

Our experts considered irradiated foods as a virtually nonexistent risk. The irradiation is done to kill bacteria and extend shelf life. "It does not make food radioactive, and there is no known cancer risk," reports L. M. Glode, M.D., of the University of Colorado Cancer Center.

The bottom lines: If you still smoke, give it up; don't be shy about asking your doctor for a cancer screening; stay out of the noonday sun; consume less alcohol and fat and more fruits, vegetables and other fiber-rich foods; and, finally, stop worrying about all that other cancer stuff you read about in the newspapers.

—Steven Lally

Dangerous Pleasures

When is too much really too much?
Here's a party pooper's guide to the dangers
lurking in life's little pleasures.

•••••••••••••••••••••••

THERE REALLY *CAN* be too much of a good thing. Not just too much money, which would surely spoil us (or so our bosses keep pointing out), but too much of normal, everyday pleasures like exercise, sleep, even water. How much is too much? In most cases *a lot*, but for those people who just never know when to stop, *Men's Health* has prepared this guide.

ALCOHOL

Within 60 minutes of downing three or more alcoholic drinks, glasses of wine or bottles of beer, your blood alcohol level can top 0.10. That's enough to get you busted for Driving While Intoxicated in most states. Twenty-five drinks in an hour can kill you, a fact that has been tragically verified at college fraternity parties over the years. The overdose of alcohol shuts down your central nervous system to the point where your brain stops sending out signals reminding you to breathe.

CAFFEINE

Caffeine is strong stuff. The amount in five or six cups of coffee—or 12 cans of cola—can make you anxious, restless, jittery. Forty cups can create symptoms that mimic severe mental illness or even a heart attack.

CARROTS

Eating more than five to six carrots per day for several months can turn your skin orange. The harmless discoloration is caused by orange pigment from the beta-carotene in the carrots and disappears once you reduce your intake. Although the problem may not help you make any new friends, it's not dangerous: You'd have to eat about 318,000 carrots to get a toxic dose of beta-carotene.

CREDIT CARDS

Carrying a wallet stuffed with too many credit cards can cause an irritation of the nerve that runs down the buttocks into the thigh, a condition doctors refer to as *creditcarditis*.

FIBER

It's hard to overdose on dietary fiber, since you'd tend to start feeling very full before you reached the danger zone. If you could manage to eat six bowls of high-fiber cereal at one sitting, you'd probably wind up with a bad stomachache from all those carbohydrates fermenting in your gut.

Fiber pills used for weight loss are another story. Some doctors have reported cases, albeit rare ones, of blocked esophagi from fiber pills expanding as patients swallowed them.

HEAT

Exercising vigorously in 90°F heat can raise your body temperature to 103° or higher, causing headaches and difficulty breathing. It's not a good idea to exercise outdoors on very hot days. If you must, drink about a half a glass of water every 10 to 15 minutes while you're working out.

HOT TUBBING

It's risky to drink liquor while you're in a hot tub because alcohol inhibits the body's temperature-regulation system. The hot water could raise your body temperature to a dangerous level and even cause your blood pressure to plunge. Should that happen, you could pass out and drown.

MUSIC

Over time, loud music destroys the tiny hairs in the ear canal that register sound waves. The louder the music, the less time this takes. For example, sitting in front of a wall of amplifiers at a rock concert for two hours is enough to do some permanent damage to your hearing.

PLAYING POOL

Playing pool for eight hours straight can produce a sharp pain in your cue-pushing shoulder. Apparently the syndrome is caused by the extension and rotation of the shoulder required by the game—an action that can compress veins of the upper chest against the first rib, causing a pain-producing blood clot.

PUSH-UPS

Doing as few as 20 to 30 push-ups a day on a hard surface may cause "push-up palsy," a numbness of the hand caused by pinching the nerve that runs through the palm. If you do a lot of push-ups, get yourself a padded mat.

SALT

Your body needs a mere 500 milligrams of salt—$\frac{1}{16}$ teaspoon—per day. You can get that in a cup of instant soup or a few handfuls of honey-roasted peanuts. The average American man eats 20 times that amount. When you begin to approach 20 to 30 grams per day (which, incidentally, is what the average Japanese consumes), you get to a level that may put you at risk for high blood pressure, arterial damage and even stroke.

SEX

We're happy to report that you can't have too much sex. Even the party poopers can't find anything wrong with overindulging here. In fact, the chances of dying in the act are so slim as to be nearly nonexistent. In a study of 5,550 men who died suddenly, only 34 of them perished during sex.

SLEEP

Sleeping more than ten hours nightly may shorten your life. A study of a million adults found that the mortality rate for long sleepers was 1½ to 2 times greater than the rate for people who slept seven to eight hours. Major causes of death were heart disease, cancer and suicide.

SODA

Six to seven cans of regular *or* diet soda daily can wreak havoc on your teeth. It's not just the sugar but also citric and phosphoric acids, commonly used flavor enhancers, that are to blame. The soda's acidity will, over time, erode tooth enamel.

SPINACH

Eating more than three cups of spinach a week may weaken your bones. Researchers found that a compound called *oxalate* in spinach blocks absorption of calcium, which in turn may result in weak, fracture-prone bones when you hit your later years.

TELEPHONING

For those with sensitive skin, eight hours on the telephone can lead to *listening-in dermatitis*, an irritation of the skin on the cheeks. The constant friction between the phone and the skin combined with perspiration and dirt from hands and the telephone receiver provides a healthy breeding ground for bacteria. The rash is common among telephone salesmen (and probably serves them right).

TOOTHBRUSHING

Too-vigorous brushing can lacerate the gum tissue and cause bleeding. Repeated rough teeth-cleaning will permanently wear away enamel and cause gums to recede. To brush properly, hold your toothbrush with your fingers rather than in your fist. Start by placing the brush just below the gum line. Then brush down on upper teeth, up on lower teeth. Always use a brush labeled "soft."

VACATION

Yes, you can get too much vacation, especially if you're a Type A. Allen Elkin, Ph.D., director of the Stress Management and Counseling Center in New York, tells us that most men begin to crave stimulation as they approach two weeks of a very relaxing vacation. If they don't get it, then the lack of stimulation creates the kind of stress they were often fleeing from in the first place. "You'll develop symptoms of stress—tension, headache, in some it's fatigue. You actually burn out from vacation," says Dr. Elkin.

VITAMIN A

A dose of 50,000 international units of vitamin A is toxic to humans. Several early Arctic explorers learned this lesson the hard way when they killed polar bears and ate the livers. Polar bears ingest huge quantities of fish, and *millions* of units of vitamin A are concentrated in their livers. The explorers developed drowsiness, irritability, headache and vomiting. A few days later, their skin began to peel off. The fact that only some lived to tell the tale proves that too much vitamin A can kill.

WATER

The typical man at rest needs about 1½ to 2 quarts of water a day (about six to eight glasses). Fifteen to 20 quarts in a day could potentially overwhelm the kidneys' ability to excrete the liquid, resulting in water intoxication. Symptoms include nausea, lightheadedness and even seizures. In severe cases, this can be fatal.

—*S. Peter Davidson*

Significant Symptoms

Forget about laughing through your discomfort.
There's no gain in some pains. If you have one of
these 25, take it to the doctor—now!

••••••••••••••••••••••

WE MEN ARE NO strangers to pain. In fact, statistics show we are far more likely than women to be victims of chest, back, abdominal and sports-related pain. Doctors say the majority of our aches and pains are best treated with rest, a couple of aspirin, an antacid or an ice pack. But, being doctors, they like to remind us that there are some pains we need their help with.

Usually those things are...well, painfully obvious. "If you feel like you've been hit by a sledgehammer, then that's a good sign that you better get to a doctor," says William Ruderman, M.D., chairman of the Department of Gastroenterology at the Cleveland Clinic Florida.

But sometimes even light taps can be a warning sign of something serious. Appendicitis, for example, usually starts with a dull ache below the navel before it intensifies. And even mild chest discomfort can sometimes be associated with heart problems.

Here's a rundown of pains you should never ignore.

HEAD

■ A headache that's accompanied by a stiff neck, lethargy, sensitivity to light or sound, nausea or vomiting. "Eighty-five to 90 percent of all headaches don't require medical attention, but when the pain persists for more than a day, recurs frequently, or is very severe or associated with telltale symptoms, then it's time to consult a physician," says Richard Lederman, M.D., Ph.D., staff neurologist at the Cleveland Clinic Foundation.

Possible problems: Encephalitis, meningitis, tumor.

• •

Safe Foods in Foreign Countries

The top health complaint of tourists abroad is traveler's diarrhea, also known as the Aztec Two-Step, Shanghai Shindig and Moscow A-Go-Go. *Patient Care* magazine offers tips to sidestep these dances.

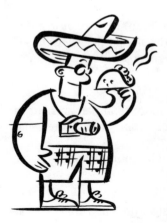

• Safe foods are steaming hot (not merely cooked), highly acidic (like citrus), dry (like breads) or very sugary (jellies and syrups).
• Unsafe foods are anything moist that sits at room temperature (sauces, salads and buffet items).
• Safe drinks include wine, bottled carbonated drinks and (steaming hot) coffee and tea. Untreated water is an invitation to boogie.

- Any head pain associated with an injury or trauma that left you disoriented or unconscious. "It's not uncommon for a person to get right up after being knocked out, only to have problems arise down the road," says Lyle Micheli, M.D., associate professor of orthopedics at Harvard University and past president of the American College of Sports Medicine. "Getting checked out right away can minimize the damage."

    Possible problems: Concussion, skull fracture.

EARS

- Ache in one or both ears, accompanied by hearing loss or discharge. The tricky part is that many times people feel better the minute their ears start to drain, according to Jerome Goldstein, M.D., executive vice-president of the American Academy of Otolaryngology–Head and Neck Surgery. "But the draining is *not* a sign that things are taking care of themselves."

    Possible problems: Infection, ruptured eardrum, damage to bones or nerves of inner ear.

- Severe pain, especially if associated with difficulty swallowing or breathing, or accompanied by fever and chills.

    Possible problems: Infection of ears or throat, tumor in the throat or mouth.

- Ringing that won't go away.

    Possible problems: Wax buildup, high or low blood pressure, drug allergy, Meniere's disease (a disorder caused by damage to the delicate structures deep inside the ear).

EYES

- Pain in one or both eyes, lasting more than half an hour or accompanied by blurred or impaired vision or extreme sensitivity to light.

    Possible problems: Infection, glaucoma, corneal scratch.

NECK

- Sore throat that gets progressively worse and makes swallowing or breathing difficult, especially if accompanied by tenderness in the neck or a fever lasting more than 48 hours. "Sore throats are usually part of the common cold, but when they start getting worse after several days or they make swallowing difficult, it's time for a doctor to have a look," says Dr. Goldstein.

Possible problems: Infection of throat, such as strep throat, or epiglottitis (inflammation of the epiglottis).

CHEST

▪ Sudden, severe pain that lasts more than five minutes; pain that gets worse with exertion, is accompanied by a tightening or pressure in the chest and shortness of breath, or radiates to the jaw, neck or arms.

Possible problems: Heart attack, angina, inflammation or infection of heart muscle.

ABDOMEN

▪ Severe pain that doesn't abate within an hour and isn't relieved by antacids. Tenderness around the site of the pain. Accompanying recurrent diarrhea or flulike symptoms such as fever, chills, nausea or vomiting.

Possible problems: Appendicitis, diverticulitis (infection of the wall of the colon or the area around the colon), gallstones, intestinal obstruction.

▪ Less severe, persistent ache lasting more than a few days and accompanied by flulike symptoms, weight loss, diarrhea or rectal bleeding.

Possible problems: Peptic ulcer, diverticulitis, a bowel infection.

▪ Sharp, constant stabbing on right side below the ribs, accompanied by flulike symptoms. May also be accompanied by jaundice (yellowing of the eyes and skin), light stools or dark urine.

Possible problem: Gallstone disease.

▪ Mild discomfort in right upper abdomen (under ribs) with prolonged illness and fatigue. May also be accompanied by jaundice and sometimes itching all over.

Possible problem: Hepatitis.

BACK

■ Pain that comes on suddenly following an injury to the back or neck—especially when accompanied by loss of bladder or bowel control, numbness, tingling or difficulty moving any limb.

Possible problems: Fractured vertebrae, ruptured or herniated disk.

■ Stabbing pain in the lower back or buttocks that shoots down the outside of one or both legs, especially when accompanied by numbness in the legs.

Possible problems: Ruptured or herniated disk, fractured vertebrae.

■ Dull ache in the lower back that gets progressively worse and may be accompanied by a burning sensation during urination, along with chills, fever or other flulike symptoms.

Possible problem: Kidney infection.

GENITALS

■ Stabbing pain in one or both testicles, often radiating to the groin and lower back. It may come and go or be accompanied by fever. "Don't be lulled into not seeing a doctor if the pain goes away temporarily," cautions J. Francois Eid, M.D., a urologist at New York Hospital–Cornell Medical Center.

Possible problem: Kidney stones.

■ Pain in one or both testicles that lasts for more than a few hours—especially if accompanied by a red, inflamed scrotum and flulike symptoms.

Possible problem: Epididymitis, an inflammation of the epididymus, the coiled passageway leading from the testis, in which sperm is produced.

■ Severe pain that comes on rapidly, occurs in only one testicle and radiates to the groin and lower abdomen. "This needs immediate attention to prevent the possibility of losing the testicle," says Dr. Eid.

Possible problem: Testicular torsion, a condition in which the testicle twists on itself, cutting off its blood supply.

■ Ache or burning that occurs during urination or intercourse, especially if accompanied by an unusual discharge or blood.

"One incident of bleeding or unusual discharge merits a trip to the doctor," advises Dr. Eid.

Possible problems: Bladder infection, prostate inflammation, sexually transmitted disease.

■ Testicle that's tender to the touch or feels harder than usual or uneven.

Possible problem: Testicular cancer, which is 90 percent curable if discovered early.

SKIN

■ Any sore that doesn't heal within a week, bleeds, changes color, is multicolored or has irregular borders.

Possible problem: Skin cancer.

■ Pain from a sting or bite that's accompanied by progressive swelling, difficulty breathing, fever, nausea or vomiting.

Possible problem: Severe allergic reaction to an insect's sting or venom, which can sometimes be fatal.

BONES, JOINTS AND MUSCLES

■ Severe pain accompanied by a heavy swelling, loss of normal motion, black-and-blue discoloration or a misshaping of the limb. "Even a trained eye may not always be able to tell if a bone is broken or not without an x-ray," comments Dr. Micheli.

Possible problems: Fracture, severe sprain or torn muscle, ligament or tendon.

■ Extreme pain in a joint, especially if accompanied by fever or rash. "Joint injuries are usually more severe than muscle or tendon injuries, and these frequently require attention," says Peter Bruno, M.D., internist for the New York Knicks.

Possible problems: Infection, fracture, torn ligament or cartilage.

■ Severe pain at the base of either calf, accompanied by the inability to rise up onto your toes.

Possible problem: Severely strained or ruptured Achilles tendon.

■ Nagging pain that's intensified over the course of a week or two. "Be especially wary of an overuse injury if the pain gets worse or comes on earlier each time you exercise," says Dr. Micheli.

Possible problems: Stress fracture, muscle strain or tear, tendinitis.

—Dan Bensimhon

A Test in Time

Having a million-dollar portfolio and a hundred-dollar body doesn't make sense. Here's a guide to taking yourself in for preventive maintenance.

••••••••••••••••••••••

TAKE CARE OF A MACHINE while it's running well, and it'll keep running well. Men know that. We change the oil in the car every 3,000 miles and schedule a maintenance service for the home heating system every fall. Unfortunately, when it comes to our bodies (our most important possession of all), we tend to be much less responsible. We avoid doctors, ignore symptoms and go to work when we're sick, in the firm belief that whatever ails us will soon pass.

Sometimes it does. But sometimes it doesn't, and medical experts say our stoic attitude toward our health is killing us. Women live an average of six years longer than we do, and many believe part of the difference has to do with the fact that women are much more willing to go to their doctors for routine checkups.

So let's put this thing in a man's terms. Think of getting physical exams as a financial investment in your future, just like putting money in a retirement account. "If you are thinking at all about retirement some day, then you have to think about the shape you're going to be in when you get there," says James Hotz, M.D., a preventive-medicine specialist at the Community Health Care Clinic in Albany, Georgia. "Having a million-dollar portfolio and a hundred-dollar body doesn't make sense."

Dr. Hotz has devised a strategy that may allow men to maintain a longer, healthier life—and the best part about the plan is that it doesn't require a lot of time in a doctor's office. While the practice of medicine is increasingly high-tech, complicated and expensive, Dr. Hotz says the art of health maintenance has become surprisingly simple and doesn't have to cost a lot of money. Studies conducted independently by Dr. Hotz and others recently reviewed by the American Academy of Family Physicians (AAFP) arrive at similar conclusions for assuring longevity: After having one comprehensive baseline physical examination, a process that takes about one hour, you need only see a doctor every couple of years for 10 or 15 minutes. And despite the array of expensive diagnostic tests that

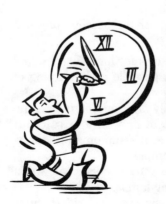

Free Time

Just how many years of life do you gain by bringing certain risk factors under control? Harvard researchers calculated that a 35-year-old man who's in danger of getting heart disease can gain:

■ **4.2 years by reducing his cholesterol level to 200 from 300 or more.**

■ **1.7 years by reducing cholesterol to 200 from 240 to 299.**

■ **2.3 years by quitting smoking.**

■ **5.3 years by bringing diastolic blood pressure down to 88 from 105 or more.**

■ **1.7 years by slimming to ideal weight from 30 percent or more above ideal.**

have been developed, only a few simple ones are actually recommended for the average man on a routine basis.

THE BASELINE PHYSICAL

This is where it all starts, a one-hour exam where you go through a battery of tests to see what kind of shape you're in and what kind of risk you're at for heart disease, cancer and lung disease. You and your doctor will then use the information obtained from your tests to tailor a health maintenance plan that fits your particular needs.

Expect the average baseline physical to cost about $250. If you have medical insurance through a health maintenance organization (HMO), it will probably pick up the entire tab. If you have health coverage through one of the major insurers, you may have to pay all or part of the bill unless the exam is ordered by your employer.

The exam will include several laboratory tests (see below), a digital or ultrasound rectal exam to look for the presence of nodules that signal prostate cancer, and a further look into your colon with a special flexible viewer, called a sigmoidoscope, to search for precancerous polyps.

Many doctors today will also provide counseling on avoiding sexually transmitted diseases, including AIDS. Whether you should have an AIDS test depends on your sexual and personal history and level of concern.

Laboratory tests recommended for the baseline physical include:

▪ Urinalysis to reveal the presence of infection. This test will also identify protein in the urine, a possible early warning of kidney disease.

▪ Thyroid profile, but generally only after age 50 unless the doctor suspects a thyroid problem or wants to rule out hypothyroidism as a possible cause of symptoms of depression. This test is run from a blood sample.

▪ Chest x-ray, which simply lets you and the doctor know that you don't have any suspicious-looking lumps.

▪ Blood tests to determine your basic liver and kidney functions, blood sugar, the amount of calcium, sodium and potassium in the blood, whether you have gout or are at risk for it, and the amount of carbon dioxide in your bloodstream (a measure of how well your heart and lungs are handling oxygen).

■ Cholesterol test, which will provide a reading of your total cholesterol. Your doctor will probably pay more attention to the specific levels of LDL (the bad kind) and HDL (the good kind). Some experts believe that low HDL levels may be the most important predictor of heart disease in men.

■ Stool blood test for an early warning of colon cancer.

■ Prostatic Specific Antigen (PSA) test for prostate cancer. This optional blood test boosts the accuracy of prostate cancer detection by 34 percent over the digital rectal exam alone. It's worth doing if you're over 50.

■ Electrocardiogram to monitor heart function under different stresses. Morris Mellion, M.D., president of the AAFP, recommends the test for men over 40 and for younger men who have abnormal cholesterol or a family history of heart disease. Furthermore, he advises *anyone* who is sedentary to have an EKG done on a treadmill to determine the heart's capacity for exercise. The results can be used to develop an exercise program.

After the results of your baseline tests come back from the lab, your doctor will want to sit you down for a chat about what they say. If there are problems, he should discuss lifestyle changes you can make to improve them. "If you develop a prevention strategy around a few key health habits, you will be able to protect yourself from 80 percent of the problems that cause premature death," says Dr. Hotz.

PERIODIC EXAMINATIONS

Dr. Mellion says that once you've had your baseline physical, you only need see a doctor again every few years for a brief exam to update your health status. His easy-to-remember formula for follow-up exams is: Two visits in your twenties, three in your thirties, four in your forties and so on. (Men with chronic illnesses such as diabetes, sickle cell disease, alcoholism or renal disease will need to make more frequent appointments, as often as once a year.)

During these return visits, your individual risk factors for the major diseases are monitored and a few of the more basic and inexpensive tests you had during the baseline physical will be repeated.

Ages 20 to 39: The physical exam should consist of height, weight and blood pressure measurements, a cholesterol test, an electrocardiogram, a testicular examination and a look at the skin for signs of cancer. Smokers and heavy drinkers should also have their mouths examined for discolorations or sores that could be precancerous.

Recommendations for periodic examinations include:

- Fasting plasma glucose test to check for adult-onset diabetes if you are overweight or have any family history of diabetes.
- Hearing test if you are in a job where you are routinely exposed to excessive noise.
- HIV test if you are concerned about exposure to the virus or are in a high-risk group for infection.
- Tetanus-diphtheria booster every ten years.
- Pneumococcal vaccine (to prevent pneumonia) and a flu shot if you have a chronic health condition like diabetes or an illness that depresses the immune system.
- Measles-mumps-rubella vaccine if you were born after 1956 and you lack evidence of immunity to measles.

Additionally, you and your doctor should continue the discussion you had at the time of your baseline physical about diet, physical activity, tobacco, alcohol and drug use, sexual practices and how to perform a testicular self-examination for nodules.

Ages 40 to 64: The physical exam should again consist of height, weight and blood pressure measurements. The doctor will also examine your skin and the inside of your mouth for precancerous signs and perform the digital rectal exam. If you have a family history of stroke or heart disease, he will also listen to the carotid artery for signs of blockage.

The laboratory tests are the same as for the 20- to 40-year-old group but also include:

- Fecal blood test and sigmoidoscopy if you are over age 50 with a family history of colorectal cancer, or a fecal blood test and colonoscopy if you have a family history of colon polyps.

■ Electrocardiogram if you have two or more risk factors for heart disease (such as smoking, obesity or high cholesterol) or if you are sedentary and want to begin an exercise program.

Your discussion should again include diet, exercise, tobacco, alcohol and drug use, sexual practices and family history of disease. Men who work outdoors or have increased exposure to sunlight should discuss using sunscreen to avoid skin cancers, and men with risk factors for heart attacks should discuss beginning aspirin therapy as a preventive measure.

Dental examinations and teeth cleaning are recommended for everyone at least once a year; some insurance carriers will pay for two cleanings a year. Eye exams are recommended about every two years.

—Tim Friend

Get It Down,
Keep It Down

16 off-the-cuff tips for keeping your blood pressure down where it belongs—all day.

●●●●●●●●●●●●●●●●●●●●●●

A WHILE AGO, I went to my doctor for a complete physical. I knew it was going to take some time, so I allocated a full hour. (Ha!) The receptionist took my name and pointed to a vacant chair. I picked up a month-old issue of *Time* magazine and sat down to wait. I finished the magazine, then another. The receptionist pretended I wasn't there. When my entire hour was almost up, I was finally escorted into a back room and told to strip to my shorts. Now, with no magazines to read and a cold draft blowing on my legs, I waited some more.

Some time later, the doctor breezed in. "How are you doing?" he asked, getting down to business by strapping a blood pressure cuff around my arm. "Fine," I said through clenched teeth, although what I really wanted to say was, "How would *you* be doing if some arrogant jerk kept you waiting more than a hour for an appointment that was scheduled months ago?"

"Hmmm," he muttered to himself as he took my blood pressure reading. "Do you use a lot of salt?"

No, I don't use a lot of salt. And I don't smoke. And never before, or since, has my blood pressure reading been that high. What I experienced that day is known as a spike, a short-term jump in blood pressure. Spikes can be caused by a multitude of things, including being pissed off.

A surge here or there is not dangerous for a healthy person. "But," says Kenneth H. Cooper, M.D., president and founder of the Aerobics Research Center in Dallas, "in people with underlying hypertension, coronary artery disease or some weakness in vessels, excessive spikes throughout the day may become a problem." In fact, they may make the condition worse and could trigger a heart attack.

In contrast to spikes are the factors that push blood pressure up more slowly, but keep it high—things like eating salty foods, drinking to excess and smoking. Ultimately you want to avoid both kinds of high blood pressure because men with hypertension are seven times more likely to have a stroke and four times more likely to have a heart attack.

Controlling high blood pressure without drugs isn't easy, and you shouldn't even try until you've discussed it with your doctor (who I hope won't *give* you high blood pressure like mine did). But it's a worthy effort. Drugs prescribed to treat hypertension are strong medicine, with common side effects, such as impotence, depression and chronic fatigue.

These tips aren't meant to be a complete program for lowering blood pressure, but they are proven techniques that can help. Work as many as you can into your life and you should see some very positive results.

1. Tell the truth. As I discovered in my doctor's examining room, blood pressure tends to spike when you lie. That's because fibbing requires your brain to work harder, according to David Robertson, M.D., director of the Clinical Research Center at the Vanderbilt University School of Medicine. "When you lie, you have to think about the truth, then manufacture something different from the truth." It's hard work. Stressful too, since there's the potential for being found out.

2. If you don't drink coffee, don't start. For some reason caffeine tends to boost blood pressure in people who don't drink it very often. In one study, bus drivers were given the equivalent of one to two cups of coffee. Those who rarely drank coffee had a surge of over five points in their blood pressure readings.

3. Rent *Annie Hall.* Or any other movie that makes you laugh. A good chuckle relaxes your body and may release endorphins, the brain's natural stress-reducing chemicals.

4. Get a dog. Having a pet is a calming influence. The minute you start talking to or petting any animal, blood pressure drops a little and stays down as long as you maintain the contact. One study even found that people who watched tropical fish in an aquarium had a measurable, if temporary, dip in blood pressure.

● ●

Here's Looking through You

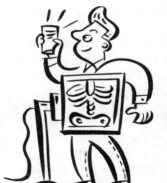

Downing a glass of orange juice or taking some vitamin C may protect you from low-level radiation like the kind you get from an x-ray. Lab mice that were fed orange juice or injected with vitamin C and then exposed to radiation showed half as much damage from rays as mice that were not fed orange juice. According to researchers, vitamin C neutralizes cell-damaging particles (called free radicals) produced in the body when it's exposed to radiation.

5. Don't shout. Simply avoiding loud, aggressive tónes may help keep blood pressure from spiking during an argument. In a study conducted by Aron Siegman, Ph.D., professor of psychology at the University of Maryland, increasing speech rate and voice volume were linked to increasing blood pressure. "If you change your speech pattern so you speak slowly and softly, even when you're angry, you will feel less angry," says Dr. Siegman.

6. Eat in Italian restaurants. In European studies, 47 patients with mildly high blood pressure who received a daily 600-milligram dose of garlic powder (roughly three to four cloves' worth) showed an average drop in blood pressure of around 11 percent.

7. Order the fish. Omega-3 fatty acids, found in ocean fish such as mackerel, tuna and salmon, may help counteract hypertension, according to a number of studies. In one report, 16 subjects taking fish-oil supplements showed as much as a four-point drop in blood pressure. Researchers still need to establish a stronger link between fish oil and blood pressure. Meanwhile, experts recommend eating fish at least twice a week.

8. *And* the broccoli. Boosting your fiber intake is one of the most important dietary changes you can make to lower blood pressure. Experts believe that increasing your fiber to 20 grams per day not only helps lower blood pressure but also reduces cholesterol. Fruits, vegetables, whole grains and legumes all head the list of good fiber bets. If you can't get enough in your diet, ask your doctor about taking regular doses of a fiber drink like Metamucil.

9. Get into training. There's evidence that moderate weight training may be as effective as medication in lowering blood pressure. However, since lifting weights can also temporarily raise blood pressure, if you have high blood pressure or a heart problem, see a doctor before starting a program.

10. Run, walk or bike. Regular aerobic exercise not only lowers blood pressure, it can help you prevent it in the first place. "People in good shape are simply less likely to develop hypertension," says Dr. Cooper, who observed this phenomenon while monitoring the effects of exercise in 4,600 people over five years. Aerobic exercise also reduces the magnitude of short-term pressure spikes, minimizing their harm to the blood vessels.

11. Shed that potbelly. Researchers have reported dramatic drops in blood pressure after men got rid of their spare tires. In one study, 60 percent of hypertensive patients who lost weight controlled their blood pressure so successfully that they were able to stop taking medication.

12. Take C and see. Two separate studies have found that people with the highest levels of vitamin C had the lowest blood pressure—and vice versa. To add vitamin C to your diet, eat more citrus fruits, green peppers, broccoli, tomatoes, strawberries and cantaloupes. You can also take vitamin C supplements.

Other research suggests that potassium brings blood pressure numbers down. Experts recommend getting at least 2,000 milligrams of this mineral each day. One baked potato

• •

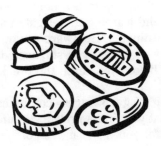

Get Your (Drug) Money's Worth

From doctors at the Mayo Clinic, here are some tips for taking medications.

■ Take medicines with a full glass of water. The drugs will be absorbed and start working faster.

■ Don't mix drugs into hot drinks. The high temperatures of coffee or tea can neutralize some drugs. And the tannin in tea can reduce absorption.

■ Check with your doctor before blending drugs with food. Crushing a pill into applesauce, for example, may make it easier for your kid to swallow but can in some cases reduce its effectiveness.

■ Also ask your doctor about taking vitamin and mineral supplements with prescribed medication. Some can alter the amount of the drug your body absorbs and the rate at which your body eliminates it.

contains 844 milligrams; one banana, 451. Other good sources include dried apricots, oranges, lima beans, Swiss chard, skim milk and chicken breast.

13. Bone up on calcium. Several studies have uncovered a link between low calcium intake and high blood pressure. And there's further evidence that upping calcium intake to normal levels can bring high blood pressure down for some individuals. If you have high blood pressure, it's a good idea to make sure you're getting at least the men's RDA (Recommended Dietary Allowance) of 800 milligrams, equal to a little less than three cups of skim milk.

14. Don't let the job kill you. In an experiment, employees ranging from stockbrokers to sanitation workers estimated the on-the-job stress they felt. They then donned portable monitors to gauge their blood pressure as they worked. Those who reported high job stress were three times as likely to have high blood pressure as those who didn't report a lot of stress.

You owe it to yourself to limit the amount of stress you feel. The best stress-busting tactics for the workplace include taking five-minute daydreaming breaks every few hours, getting out for a walk at lunchtime and learning to delegate the maddening little details to subordinates. Be aware of your body's response to stress, whether it's a tense jaw, stiff neck or headache, and catch the tension before you reach the breaking point.

15. Stay cool at home. The fight against stress continues at home. Experts recommend that you find a private 20 minutes somewhere in your day just for you. You can read or just sit quietly, but the goal is to initiate what doctors call *the relaxation response*. This is a measurable body change that includes a slowing of metabolism, heart rate, rate of breathing and blood pressure. The relaxation response dilutes anger, anxiety and depression, says Herbert Benson, M.D., associate professor of medicine at Harvard Medical School.

16. Cut back on salt. If you have high blood pressure, probably the most important thing you can do for the problem is to cut back on salt. "There's no question in my mind that sodium is the major culprit in high blood pressure," says Norman Kaplan, M.D., head of the Hypertension Division at

• •

BLOOD PRESSURE PRIMER:
WHAT THE NUMBERS MEAN

Blood pressure readings are actually a double measurement of the force of the blood against arterial walls. You need two measurements so you can tell how much pressure builds up in the arteries both as the heart beats and between beats. The high number gives a sense of the pumping force of the heart. The lower number indicates flexibility and clogging in the arteries.

The reading is usually taken by wrapping an inflatable cuff around the upper part of your arm. Air is pumped into the cuff until circulation is cut off. At this point, when a stethoscope is placed over the artery in your arm, nothing can be heard. Then the air is slowly let out of the cuff until you can hear blood begin to flow through again. This is your systolic pressure, the high number in your reading, and it's expressed in how high it would send a column of mercury in a tube. A reading of 120 millimeters is considered normal.

As air continues to be let out of the cuff, the pressure of the cuff becomes so low that the sound of the blood surging against partially closed artery walls disappears. This is the diastolic pressure, the low number. A normal reading is 80 millimeters.

Readings above 140/90 indicate hypertension. In effect, it's a sign that the heart is working extra hard to get blood through the circulatory system because of narrow or inflexible arteries or both. Over a period of time, an overworked heart becomes enlarged and less efficient. And the added pressure damages arterial walls, leading to scarring and hardening of these vessels.

• •

the University of Texas Health Science Center.

An analysis of more than 70 studies concluded that if everyone cut back on daily salt intake by three grams (about 1½ teaspoons), the incidence of stroke would be slashed by 26 percent and one kind of heart disease by 15 percent. Put another way, not salting our food could save an estimated 180,000 American lives each year.

—*Greg Gutfeld*

No More Back Pain

You can turn a bad back into a good back.
Just 15 minutes a day can give you a lifetime
of freedom from back pain.

• •

BACK EXPERTS AGREE that one of the best ways to avoid back pain is to exercise: If you keep your body flexible, strong and well conditioned, they say, you're far less likely to get a backache.

Still, simply being active isn't enough, since back pain hits active men, too. (Sports greats Joe Montana, Larry Bird, Don Mattingly, Jack Nicklaus and Mario Lemieux all have bum backs.)

If you're among the 53 percent of men who have been laid low by back pain, you know what a downright frustrating and debilitating experience it can be. You're in agony, you can't work, you can't play, you can't walk, you can't get in and out of bed on your own, let alone make love while you're there. Back pain makes weak men out of strong ones.

But you don't have to take back pain lying down. The experts are right about the significance of exercise, but it's important to get the right kind. If your fitness regimen consists of playing tennis a couple of times a week, hefting weights solely to build killer biceps and riding your bike on weekends, you qualify as active, but you aren't doing much that will help build a stronger back. To do that, you have to target your back for its own exercise program.

Despite all the scary talk you hear about blown disks and degenerating joints, the vast majority of painful back episodes are caused by muscle strain, which, among active men, usually comes from two things, says Mitch Bogdanffy, an exercise physiologist at the Texas Back Institute (TBI).

The first is demanding more of back muscles than they can handle: lifting heavy objects improperly (the familiar advice to lift with the legs, keeping the back straight and objects close to the body, is ignored with astonishing regularity) or going overboard on leisure activities such as sports and gardening.

TAKE IT EASY AT FIRST

You're particularly at risk of throwing out your back with racquet sports, golf, bowling, football, canoeing, baseball, basketball or anything requiring lots of arching, twisting and sudden starts and stops. To minimize back strain from these sports, it's best to take it easy at the start of the season or when first learning, always easing muscles in and out of activity with warm-ups, cool-downs and stretches.

A second cause of strain is weak muscles, especially in the abdomen. Strong abdominal muscles help to stabilize the lower back, the spine's most vulnerable point. Weak ones allow an exaggerated curve in the lower back, a posture that crimps muscles, nerves and disks.

One study found back-pain sufferers to have just as much back-muscle endurance as healthier people, but weaker stomach muscles. You don't have to be doing anything particularly strenuous to throw out your back if the abdominal muscles are soft—many men report being flattened by pain while bending over to tie a shoelace or pat the dog, or reaching around to grab a briefcase off the car seat. These actions by themselves don't cause the backache; they're just the straw that broke the camel's you-know-what.

"A weak belly strains the muscles that run along the lower spine," explains physical therapist and fitness author Carol Greenburg. "They are always being pulled, they are always resisting, and they simply get exhausted from the effort. Simple exhaustion can throw a muscle into spasm, a contraction that feels like a knot, hurts like the devil and won't let go for days."

If your problem is weak abdominals (which it probably is if you're not currently doing anything specific to strengthen them), boosting the muscles with exercise is the best thing you can do to protect your back.

The YMCA Healthy Back Program, a respected exercise regimen that dates back to the 1940s, devotes its strengthening exercises almost exclusively to the abdominals. In an evaluation of 233 patients who took part in the program, 82 percent found that their usual back pain either stopped or decreased significantly. Only 2.5 percent of the participants showed little or no improvement.

Specifically, here's how building strong stomach muscles can help bolster your back.

It stabilizes the spine. "The abdominal muscles and the low back muscles together form a column of muscles that must be strong all around," says Wayne Westcott, Ph.D., YMCA national strength-training consultant. When strong and balanced, these trunk muscles ease the spine's structural and weight-carrying burden. "But if one side is weak, it may put excess stress on the spine and the nerves and tissue that surround it," Dr. Westcott says.

It cuts flab. A potbelly can make spinal instability worse. "For Americans, the abdomen is exercised very little, and it's where body fat tends to migrate," says Dr. Westcott. It's a double whammy, like sending extra traffic to a congested bridge with weak supports. Something's got to give—in this case, your spine. Coupling a low-fat diet with a full exercise program that emphasizes abdominals may be as close as you can get to natural liposuction for the gut.

It eases everyday movements. A strong abdomen helps the body cope with everyday resistive activities, whether moving furniture or climbing stairs, lugging a heavy suitcase or catching a ball. "If those abdominal muscles are weak, you'll overcompensate with your back," says TBI physical therapist Paula Gilbert. "This can lead to a back sprain over and over again. You need to have these stomach and back muscles synergized—working together—or your back will not respond well after injury."

GET STRONG ALL OVER

Zeroing in on your stomach muscles makes almost no sense, however, if you neglect everything else. At the Texas Back Institute, specialists emphasize the importance of cardiovascular fitness for decreasing back pain and injury, and recommend aerobic exercise—walking, swimming, water exercises, stationary cycling—for any back-building program.

"Cardiovascular exercise lubricates the joints and stretches muscles so they're less prone to strain and tearing," says Stephen Hochschuler, M.D., surgeon and TBI cofounder. Research backs this up: A study of 1,652 firefighters found that the most cardiovascularly fit of them had ten times fewer debilitating back injuries than the least fit.

Exercise also promotes the efficient transport of oxygen to muscles, which helps healing, and boosts daily production of your body's self-made painkillers, endorphins and enkephalins.

To strengthen specific muscles that support the spine and help the back do its job, you also need to include the abdominals, the oblique muscles (running from the back of the spine to the front of the abdomen), the extensor muscles of the lower back and the leg muscles that share lifting duty.

The following routine hits them all, but especially works those abdominals. You can do the complete workout at home in less than 15 minutes.

• •

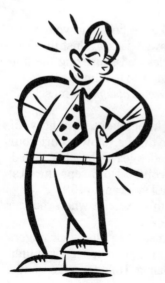

The Short Leg to Back Pain

If you have an aching back, it may be because one of your legs is shorter than the other. Even a slight inequality can cause the spine to curve to the short side when you walk or run. Eventually, the bend puts painful pressure on disks. Most people can't tell if their legs are different lengths, says researcher Steven McCaw, Ph.D., of Illinois State University: "A tailor measuring for pants is often the first to pick it up." The simplest way to correct the problem is to put a Dr. Scholl–type therapeutic insert into your shoe to give the shorter leg a lift.

First, some pointers:

■ To get the most back-boosting benefits, do the exercises three or more times a week.

■ Exercise with slow, controlled movements: Speed adds momentum, momentum carries you, and the muscles end up doing less work.

■ Avoid full sit-ups, which use only about 30 percent of the abdominal muscles, leaving the hip flexors to do most of the work. If you rise only slightly, your abdominals will do 90 percent of the work.

■ When you're performing these exercises, put something between you and the ground. A body-length mat, available at just about any sporting goods store, cushions your back much better than a cold, hard floor.

■ People with back pain can usually do light exercises. But see a doctor first if no position gives you relief, if your pain's lasted more than two weeks, if it radiates down your leg to your knee or foot, or if simple movement makes the pain worse.

Now, your routine:

Pelvic tilt. This exercise primarily strengthens abdominal muscles, but it also builds muscles in the lower back that keep it properly aligned with the pelvis.

Lie on your back, with your knees bent and your arms extended to the side. Press your lower back against the floor by tightening the abdominal muscles and squeezing the buttocks. Hold for ten seconds. Repeat five to ten times.

Partial curl. This targets the *rectus abdominis* muscles at the front of the body.

Lie on your back with your knees bent. Extend your hands straight out between your thighs. Slowly curl your upper torso until your shoulder blades leave the floor, exhaling while rising. Hold for ten seconds. Do 5 reps the first week, then increase by 5 a week until you can do 15.

Advanced curl. Move on to this exercise when you can easily do 20 partial curls.

Lie on your back, with your knees bent and your fingers lightly touching your ears. Slowly curl your upper torso until your shoulders leave the floor, exhaling. Hold for ten seconds.

• •

WHO'LL STOP THE PAIN?

Who is most likely to provide relief from back pain? An orthopedist? A neurologist? How about a neurosurgeon? The answer—at least in one survey of 492 back-pain sufferers—is none of the above.

Practitioner	Moderate to Dramatic Long-Term Relief (%)	Temporary Relief (%)
Yoga instructors	96	4
Physiatrists	86	0
Physical therapists	65	0
Acupuncturists	36	32
Chiropractors	28	28
Osteopathic physicians	28	15
Neurosurgeons	26	8
Orthopedists	23	9
Family practitioners	20	14
Massage therapists	10	63
Neurologists	4	4

• •

Start with five reps, increasing by fives as they get easy.

Twist curl. This works the obliques, or side abdominal muscles.

Lie on the floor with your knees bent. Fold your arms across your chest. Slowly curl your right shoulder off the floor toward the left knee until your left shoulder leaves floor. Hold for ten seconds, breathing deeply. Repeat, but with your left shoulder toward your right knee. Do three of each.

Spinal extension. This strengthens the lumbar extensor muscles of the lower back.

Lie face down on your stomach with your elbows bent and your fingers lightly touching your ears. Lift your upper body off the floor, exhaling. Hold for ten seconds. Do 5 reps to start, then add 2 a week until you can do 15 to 20.

Advanced spinal extension. Start this exercise when you can do 15 to 20 spinal extensions.

Use the same position as in the spinal extension, but with your arms extended straight out in front of you. Do five reps to start, increasing by twos as they become easy.

Leg extension. This strengthens the quadriceps.

Sit on a surface that allows your legs to dangle straight down from the knee without touching the ground. Wearing ankle weights, straighten one leg in a slow, controlled motion. Repeat with the other leg. The weight should be heavy enough to slightly fatigue muscles after 12 reps. Increase to 15 reps after the first week. After 2 weeks at 15 reps, boost the weight by five pounds.

If you'd like to find out more about the YMCA back program, call the National YMCA at (800) 872-9622 for information on local programs. If you have questions on specific back problems, contact the Texas Back Institute at (800) 247-2225.

—Greg Gutfeld

Part 8

LOOKING
GOOD

Through Thick
and Thin

*Are you tired of "hair today, gone tomorrow"
jokes? Well, here is some of the most comforting
hair-raising news to sprout up in years.*

••••••••••••••••••••••

BEFORE MINOXIDIL CAME ALONG, it was prudent to classify *all* baldness treatments as snake oil. The success of
Rogaine, Upjohn's minoxidil-based lotion, was a wake-up call
to entrepreneurs in medical research. It proved not only that
it's possible for a drug to grow hair (at least for some men)

but, equally important, that it's possible to get the seal of approval for a hair restorer from the Food and Drug Administration (FDA).

As the pioneer, Rogaine has had the entire hair-loss market to itself. It brought in $140 million worldwide in 1990 alone. But that figure pales in comparison to the *potential* earnings for a baldness remedy; 30 to 40 percent of all adult men are losing their hair, and most would like to do something about it.

Eager for a share of that bonanza of profits, a number of companies are competing to be next up with a baldness breakthrough. Although no new treatments are headed for pharmacy shelves immediately, some promising research is under way. Here's a progress report.

TRICOMIN

This drug is so new that some of the most knowledgeable hair-loss experts in the country haven't heard of it yet. Early tests with lab mice at the University of Wisconsin suggest that Tricomin may be able to restore lost locks, so to hasten testing in humans, the drug's maker, ProCyte Corporation of Kirkland, Washington, has taken it to France, where pretest

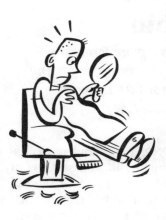

When the Barber Slips Up
That haircut seemed fine when the barber handed you the mirror, but now, the next day, it looks like a nest of snakes. Chances are your hair was cut too short. Hair that's been on the long side will sometimes spring up when cut short since there's no longer anything weighing it down. One remedy is to dump a handful of mousse or gel on it and comb everything back. If that's not your style, ask your barber to fit you in for an emergency repair job right away. As a general rule, it takes a week for a new haircut to settle.

requirements are less stringent than in the United States. Early results from the first study, just completed at the University of Rheims, show that men given high doses of Tricomin show significant regrowth of what are known as terminal hairs. "That's what you or I would call real hair, not peach fuzz," says ProCyte's vice-president of research, Gordon Dunkin, Ph.D. In some cases, results were seen in as little as one month.

Present theory holds that Tricomin causes new blood vessels to form in the scalp and boosts the pate's production of collagen, a natural protein that keeps skin supple and healthy. "Which one of these is causing hair to grow, we don't know," Dr. Dunkin admits.

On this side of the Atlantic, human trials are expected to begin soon.

AROMATASE

Some researchers believe that the future of baldness treatment lies in deactivating or blocking the male hormones in the scalp that cause the follicles (from which hairs sprout) to shut down. Theoretically, any drug that blocks the action of these hormones could control hair loss, and a number have been tried. The trick is to isolate their effects on the scalp without unsafely throwing off the hormonal balance elsewhere in the body.

In a key discovery, researchers at the University of Miami have isolated an enzyme, aromatase, that balding men are deficient in. When the enzyme is present in high-enough levels, follicles grow hair, but when there's not enough, follicles switch off. What's especially promising about this hormone is that it seems to affect skin and hair exclusively.

According to Marty Sawaya, M.D., Ph.D., an assistant professor of dermatology and leader of the research, we can expect to see successful hormone treatments for hair loss within five to ten years.

ELECTRICAL STIMULATION

Applying low-powered pulses of electrical stimulation to the scalp grew new hair or prevented hair loss in 29 of 30 men taking part in Canadian tests. The treatment consists of sitting under a helmetlike hood that painlessly bathes the head with mild current for 12 minutes, twice a week. "The method sounds quackish, but the research that's being done is legitimate," says Harry Roth, M.D., clinical professor of dermatology at the University of California in San Francisco.

Because of the success of early research, a new round of trials was inaugurated at 14 sites across the United States and Canada and is just now winding down. These tests could bring the method a step closer to FDA approval, but because they're double-blind studies, not even those in charge can yet say whether they have been successful. If they have, dermatologists could conceivably be offering this treatment in their offices within a few years.

CYOCTOL

A few years ago, a study found that Cyoctol, a hormone-blocking drug stopped hair loss or grew new hair in 92 percent of men who used it as a lotion for a year. Since then, as the company was seeking corporate backing, no further clinical trials have been done. Some experts took the lack of news as a bad omen for the drug. But last year, Cyoctol's maker signed an agreement with Upjohn, the makers of Rogaine, who will continue research and development.

DIAZOXIDE

This drug's potential was discovered when patients taking it to treat hyperinsulinemia, a rare-but-deadly pancreatic disorder, began sprouting excessive body hair. Early experiments show that it can also grow hair when applied directly to the head. Ken Hashimoto, M.D., who's done research on the drug at Wayne State University School of Medicine in Detroit, Michigan, speculates that it works by dilating blood vessels in the scalp, delivering more raw material to the hair-producing machinery of the follicles.

Don't expect to see this treatment on your drugstore shelves soon. "Unfortunately, the human studies have been uncontrolled, so there is no scientific proof and no regulatory approval," says Dr. Hashimoto.

• •

THE *MEN'S HEALTH* BALD-O-METER

There are 100,000 hairs on the typical male head, and on any given day, you lose 50 to 100 of them, whether you're balding or not. If you're unsure whether the amount of hair coming out in your comb is worth worrying about, try this simple test. Grab a clump of hair and tug gently but firmly. It's normal for six or fewer hairs to come out. More than six could be an early warning that you may someday be sporting the Jack Nicholson look.

• •

The bottom line on baldness remedies? "In five to ten years, more men will have more options, and the treatments that exist will be more refined," says Douglas Altchek, M.D., assistant clinical professor of dermatology at Mt. Sinai School of Medicine in New York City.

Waiting for any of these new therapies to struggle over the mountainous federal drug-regulating bureaucracy could take more time than many balding men want to wait. The biggest advances that can make a difference to you right now have come in hair-transplantation techniques. In the past, large plugs of hair were taken from the back of the head and grafted to the bald area, sometimes leaving the patient with an artificial "doll's hair" look.

Using new techniques, doctors can work with much smaller plugs—or even single hairs—allowing them to create a softer, more natural hairline, especially when hair and skin are both light or both dark so that the contrast between them is less noticeable. The grafts are planted into small slits in the scalp, which causes less scarring and growth-impairing damage to the skin and blood vessels than do traditional methods. "These techniques are the most important developments in hair-replacement surgery in two decades," says Dowling Stough, M.D., chief of hair transplant at the Baylor Hair Research and Treatment Center in Dallas.

Time and cost are the only drawbacks. The new procedures take two to three times longer (usually about three hours for each of about four sessions) and roughly double the price to around $2,000 per session. The method works best for men who still have some hair left in the area to be regrown.

To find out more about this option or to see if you're a good candidate for minoxidil, consult a dermatologist.

—*Richard Laliberte*

New Lease on White

If flashing a high-beam smile is important to you, you're in luck. These new at-home teeth-whitening kits can put the gleam back in your grin.

• •

BY THE TIME A MAN reaches his midthirties, that blindingly white 150-watt smile he had when he was a kid has dimmed to about 75 watts or so. Even with diligent brushing, flossing and regular visits to the dental hygienist, teeth tend to yellow over the years as tiny interlacing cracks in the enamel absorb stains from coffee, tea, tobacco, wine and certain soft drinks.

It's been possible for some years now to bleach teeth back to their natural white color, but until recently that process involved three to five lengthy dental appointments (at $200 a shot) for teeth to be individually lightened. The dentist would cover your gums with a rubber guard, painstakingly apply a 30 percent hydrogen peroxide solution, Superoxol, to each tooth, and then blast it with a heat lamp to activate the bleach.

Today, in a technique some dentists are calling revolutionary, you skip most of the office visits and bleach your own teeth. You start the program with a dental appointment to make sure your gums are healthy and your teeth clean. (The 10 percent carbamide peroxide solution or gel that's used can irritate unhealthy gums and won't work effectively on teeth with a lot of plaque buildup.) The dentist takes a mold of your teeth and creates a custom mouthpiece for you to take home. Each day you apply the peroxide gel to the mouthpiece and wear it for two to four hours.

Most people begin to see results in about a week, and the process is usually complete in a month. Twelve to 18 months down the line, you can use the mouthpiece for a couple of hours just to keep the yellow at bay. Cost (including dentist visit and supplies): $150 to $500 per arch. Many people treat only the top teeth, as lowers aren't as prominent when you smile.

These dentist-supervised kits are catching on in a big way—at an American Dental Association (ADA) convention, about 90 percent of the 500 dentists attending a lecture on the subject said they were using the mouthpiece technique. Only about 2 to 3 percent said they were having problems with it.

OVER-THE-COUNTER KITS

For a much less expensive alternative, there are many over the-counter teeth whiteners. These pastes or polishes may contain weaker concentrations of some kind of peroxide agent than the dentist-supervised kits and are designed to be left on the teeth for as little as ten minutes per day.

But there's not much hard evidence on how well they work. Some patients report favorable, though unpredictable, results with mild stains. "Little research exists on the long-term safety of these products, but as yet, few problems have been reported," says Joel M. Boriskin, D.D.S., chief of the Division of Dentistry at Highland General Hospital in Oakland, California.

Still, dentists will tend to steer you away from the do-it-yourself kits. Chakwan Siew, Ph.D., head of the ADA's Department of Toxicology, warns that long-term use of hydrogen peroxide can damage chromosomes and boost the cancer-causing effects of other substances. Peroxide may also infect or damage the soft tissues of the mouth or even the interior of the tooth. (None of that is likely if you stay within the product guidelines.)

Some over-the-counter kits include their own mouth guard. But Richard Price, D.M.D., a consumer advisor for the ADA, warns that an ill-fitting mouth guard could actually hold the bleach against the gums and burn them—precisely the problem it is designed to prevent. The mouth guard needs to be custom fitted and trimmed, he says—"One size does not fit all."

But several manufacturers of at-home bleaching kits, notably EpiSmile and Den-Mat (makers of the Rembrandt Lighten system), are cooperating with the ADA. In a study reported in the *Journal of Esthetic Dentistry,* the Rembrandt system produced a "definite improvement relative to the shade of the treated teeth" in 43 patients and left "no sensitivity or unpleasant aftertaste."

IN THE DENTIST'S OFFICE

A follow-up study found no complications and in some cases an *improvement* in the condition of the gums.

If bleaching isn't doing the trick for you or isn't appropriate, consider these teeth-whitening options.

Bonding. In this procedure, your teeth are covered with a pastelike bonding material that is hardened under a high-intensity light. It lasts from three to eight years. Cost: $200 to $500 per tooth.

Veneers. The front of the tooth is painted with adhesive, then an ultrathin porcelain veneer is pressed into place. At $275 to $850 per tooth, this is more expensive than composite bonding, but veneers can last for ten years or more.

Crowns. Capping a tooth with a crown may be the only option for severe stains. Crowns require more work and are more expensive than veneers. They last 10 to 12 years. Cost: $445 to $1,000 per tooth.

—*Ron Heitzgebot*

● ●

Workers of the World, Dress Up!

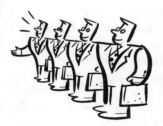

Most office workers favor dress codes, according to a Gallup Poll of 500 managers and office workers. Despite the cost and discomfort of "proper business attire," two out of three workers think it's "very" or "fairly" important to have a corporate dress code.

Optical Options

*Confused by all the styles and choices when
you shop for eyeglasses? Here's a buyer's guide
to help you see your way clear.*

••••••••••••••••••••••

LET ME DESCRIBE my typical visit to an eyeglass store. I
step through the door of Lens Land or Optical World or whatever and am immediately confronted by four million sets of
frames hanging on invisible racks. I'm still trying to figure out
which are the men's and which are the women's when an
attractive woman approaches and asks if I need help.

"Uh, yes," I reply. "I need some new glasses."

"Great. Are you interested in metal frames or plastic?
Single vision or bifocals? Glass or polycarbonate lenses?
Scratch-resistant coating? Antireflective tint? UV filtering?"

At this point I reach for my checkbook and turn my decisions completely over to the salesperson. A few weeks later I
stop back to pick up my glasses and return home, whereupon
my girlfriend says something like, "Hmmm. New glasses. Um,
maybe you should take me with you next time you get new
frames."

Sound at all familiar?

These days, buying prescription eyeglasses is a real challenge. You're faced with considerable (and often confusing)
options on everything from the size of the frames to the types
of lenses and what they're coated with. At least when you shop
for a car, you get to take a test drive and kick the tires. With
glasses, you're stuck with the choices you make up front.

I've found that shopping for eyeglasses is a lot easier
when you're armed with some basic information. Whether you
get your next pair from a private optician or optometrist or at
that flashy optical chain at the mall, it pays to do a little home-
work. To help, I've assembled a summary of what's out there
in vision wear, including materials, coatings and lenses. Take a
look.

LENS MATERIAL

Glass. All eyeglasses used to have glass lenses, and it remains a popular material, mainly because it provides a hard, scratch-resistant surface. Its big drawback is its weight.

"If you have a high-powered prescription, wearing thick glass lenses may be too much weight for your nose to bear," says Irving Bennett, O.D., of the American Optometric Association.

Plastic. "Plastic lenses are safer, more impact-resistant and much lighter than glass, giving you a more comfortable fit," says Richard Morgenthal, of Morgenthal-Frederics Opticians, in New York City. When larger lenses became fashionable, lightweight plastic came to dominate the market. However, plastic lenses are much more vulnerable to scratches than glass. "You should always get a scratch-resistant coating on your plastic lens," says Dr. Bennett. Some places may offer the coating as standard with plastic lenses.

Polycarbonate plastic. These lenses are made of a lighter but tougher plastic, distinctive enough that eye-care specialists classify them in a separate category. Polycarbonate-plastic lenses were first introduced as virtually unbreakable, with people slamming hammers on them to demonstrate the lenses' strength. Experts say most people don't really need this kind of protection. Polycarbonate is recommended for children younger than 16 and anyone who plays contact sports or who works in a hazardous industry. Polycarbonate, although strong, is still prone to scratching, so if you choose it, get the scratch-resistant coating.

COATINGS AND FILTERS

While coatings are becoming an increasingly popular extra, the real need for some may be overstated. Also, they don't last forever. Most opticians agree that if you take really good care of coated lenses, clean them carefully and don't wipe them on your shirttail, coatings can last a few years.

Scratch-resistant coatings. As the name implies, these don't make plastic lenses scratch*proof*, but they do protect against the hairline scratches that occur from normal cleaning and handling. They won't prevent damage from more serious indiscretions such as throwing your glasses on the car dash, dropping them on the sidewalk or putting them in the same pocket as your car keys.

If you buy glass lenses, you won't need this coating. It is necessary for polycarbonate lenses and recommended for plastic ones.

Tints. Tints, especially the colors brown, green and gray, may help give you clearer vision in sunlight. If you opt for a tint, make sure it's not so dark that it impairs your vision indoors.

UV filters. Most glasses these days already come with built-in protection from ultraviolet rays. "The majority of UV light is filtered by any glass or plastic material," says H. Jay Wisnicki, M.D., director of ophthalmology at Beth Israel Medical Center in New York City. "The extra coatings may not be that important." Take the windows of your car, for example. If you drive with your arm against the window in the blistering sun, it won't get burned. But hang it out the window and you may get a truck-driver's tan. That's the kind of protection you get with most glass. If you want extra peace of mind, you can opt for the coating, but it's not really needed, says Dr. Wisnicki.

As for UV rays seeping from computers, that threat too may be exaggerated. "The amount of UV light that comes from a computer is very small and shouldn't be regarded as a problem," says Dr. Wisnicki. The American Academy of Ophthalmology considers video display terminals (VDTs) to be completely safe, presenting no hazard to the eye.

Photochromic lenses. Photochromics, lenses that change from clear to dark, may be a convenient choice for someone whose job requires a combination of indoor and out-door work. Different brands go from light when indoors to varying degrees of darkness when outside. "They shouldn't be used for driving, however, because the lenses need UV light to stimulate darkening, and UV light is blocked by windshield glass," says Morgenthal.

If you have photochromics, here's a tip to make them work better: "If you consistently store these lenses overnight in the refrigerator, they'll respond quicker to light and get darker," says Morgenthal.

Antireflective coatings. These coatings—made from the same material used to coat camera lenses and binoculars—can block out reflected glare. Consider one if you do a lot of night driving—it virtually eliminates the starburst effect you get from oncoming headlights. It can also cut glare from other types of lighting.

One of the drawbacks of antiglare coating, though, is a tendency to smudge. You'll have to take extra care to keep your lenses clean. Dr. Wisnicki, who owns a pair, agrees, saying, "The dirt seems to show up more." There's a new Teflon-like coating out now, though, that goes over the antiglare coating and may make the lenses easier to care for.

SPECIAL LENSES

High-index lenses. These are simply denser lenses with a higher power of refraction, meaning they can bend more light than standard-index glasses can, so less material is needed to do the job. Thus the lenses can be thinner and lighter.

They're a must for anyone who needs strong prescription glasses but who doesn't want the Coke-bottle look.

Bifocals. Previously, when it came to combating presbyopia (the gradual decline in the eye lens's ability to focus on nearby objects), one could turn only to bifocals. With them, only two distances mattered—near and far. There was no in-between. Now new lenses offer effective alternatives to the split-level world of bifocal vision, some that erase the bifocals' age-giveaway lines while giving sharp vision at different distances.

Trifocals. Bifocals have "near" and "far" covered. Trifocals offer an extra area of power on the lens to bridge the near and far. The visual breakdown when looking through a common trifocal lens goes like this: far distance up top, medium distance in the middle and close at the bottom.

Trifocals aren't for everyone. "Some people may not be able to get used to the 'image jumps' that occur when switching from one segment to the next," says Richard E. Lippman, O.D., director of the Division of Ophthalmic Devices for the Food and Drug Administration. It's a problem encountered with bifocals and can become more troublesome in a trifocal with the extra segment, he says.

Progressive-addition lenses. If the bifocal or trifocal is the stairway of lenses, then a progressive bifocal lens is the smooth ramp. Gone are the abrupt jumps in vision power. You see a blended transition from one segment of vision to the next, closely mimicking good natural vision.

The most obvious benefit the progressive-addition lenses have over bifocals is the absence of the age-telling demarcation lines—the lines can't be seen because the focal powers blend into each other.

Ready-to-wears. You've seen them in neat racks at the pharmacy—simple reading glasses that cost about $12 a pair. They're inexpensive, but are they a good idea for poor eyesight?

"When it comes to reading newspapers or other types of short-term reading, these glasses are harmless," says Dr. Lippman. However, he adds a caveat: "Because these lenses come in basic, fixed corrections, with no gradual increments in between, you're really guessing at your prescription when you pick one up," he says. "They shouldn't keep you from getting regular checkups to determine what kind of correction you need and to see if there's any underlying illness behind the vision change."

PRICING

Every company that sells eyeglasses has its own pricing system. Some charge the same for plastic and glass lenses, while others may charge more for one than the other. Some offer options like free tints, while others tack on $15 to $30 extra. So what do you do and where do you start?

"Be wary of come-ons and promotions," warns Dr. Bennett. Those buy-one-pair-get-one-free spiels, for example. "They usually involve a discontinued product," he says. "It'll be a naked lens with no frills, coatings or treatments—and they may nail you on that."

Don't be surprised if you find that the major chains—the ones found most frequently at malls—charge a little more. "Having a sales force, paying higher rent and using expensive machinery makes their overhead higher, so it's understandable that their prices are higher," says Dr. Bennett.

The key, then, is to get an idea of what you want beforehand and call around. If you feel you're getting a sales pitch instead of honest advice, skip the place. Compare identical products. A plastic lens with a scratch-resistant coating and a gray tint may be priced differently from one with high index and antiglare coating.

Ask for itemized prices for all the lenses and coatings, and be sure you're comparing the same brands. And don't forget money-back guarantees. Many brands of lenses and coatings carry them. It's up to you to ask.

I've found, or rather my girlfriend has reminded me, that it's hard to judge for yourself what kind of frames look best on your face. My favorite glasses are some snazzy oval tortoiseshells. I see them on men all the time and I like the way they look. But on me, according to my significant other, they look stupid.

If you're not sure what kind of frames you look best in, bring along a friend to help you decide. Don't rely on the salesperson. She's probably been asked that question 200 times that day and is beyond rational judgment.

—*Greg Gutfeld*

Timely Contacts

Extended-wear contact lenses are great, as long as you don't take the "extended" part too literally. How long can you leave your new lenses in?

••••••••••••••••••••••

IF YOU SLEEP WITH your extended-wear contact lenses in, you're 10 to 15 times more likely to develop a painful and potentially serious eye condition called *ulcerative keratitis* than people who take their lenses out every night, reports a team of ophthalmologists from the Massachusetts Eye and Ear Infirmary and Harvard Medical School.

"I wouldn't tell most people that they should never sleep with their contact lenses in, but they certainly should never do it for more than seven days," warns Johanna M. Seddon, M.D., one of the researchers.

Ulcerative keratitis occurs when an abrasion in the cornea, the clear covering of the eye, allows bacteria to enter and cause an infection. Untreated, it can impair sight by causing scar tissue to form, blocking part of the field of vision.

Until about a decade ago, virtually all cases of ulcerative keratitis occurred in eyes that were already predisposed somehow to such damage, says Dr. Seddon. But as soft contact lenses became popular, eye doctors began seeing it in eyes that were otherwise healthy. Contact lenses now account for about 30 percent of the cases. And most of those, says Dr. Seddon, can be blamed on excessive overnight lens wearing.

Can You Skinny Dip with Your Contacts?

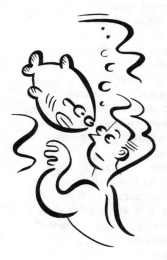

It's okay to swim with your contact lenses in, says an article in *The Physician and Sportsmedicine,* but heed these safety tips.

■ After swimming anywhere—even in chlorinated pools—always remove your contacts and clean them with an antibacterial cleaner.

■ Pool water and lake water cause soft lenses to dry out and stick to your eyes. To keep from scratching your eyes as you peel off the lenses, wait about a half hour after swimming, or wet them first with saline solution.

■ Wearing contacts won't help you see better underwater; water distorts the prescription completely. So wear prescription goggles.

Exactly how is still unknown. But there are some clues. "Contact lenses can cause tiny injuries to the cornea, and they also reduce the amount of oxygen that reaches it," she says. "Both factors could let bacteria and other harmful organisms establish themselves."

It turns out that extended-wear lens users aren't the only people who go to bed without taking out their contacts. In the Harvard study, the doctors found a surprising number of *daily*-wear lens users did. And as you might expect, they too had an increased incidence of ulcerative keratitis.

"I have to emphasize that it's not contact lenses that are the risk factor here," says Dr. Seddon. "The risky thing is leaving them in for several days in a row."

RULES TO LIVE BY

When extended-wear contacts came on the market, the Food and Drug Administration allowed manufacturers to say they could be left in for 30 days between cleanings. Partly as a

• •

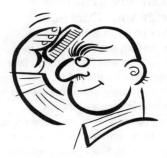

Hair in All the Wrong Places

As we age, hair begins to fall out of places where we want it and begins growing where we don't want it. Whatever the cause, the solution is to trim the unwanted hair.
Fredric Haberman, M.D., clinical instructor of medicine at Albert Einstein College of Medicine, suggests the following methods.

■ Trim eyebrow hair with a fine, small comb and scissors.

■ Prune hair off the edges of your ears with a special electric clipper (available at drugstores) that comes with its own ear-protecting safety shield.

■ Snip away hair from the inside of ears and nose with a manual rotary clipper (also available at drugstores). But be extra careful inside the ears and nose, as you could injure these delicate areas, says Dr. Haberman.

result of the new study, the month is now down to 7 days. Some eye doctors say it should be shortened even more. Dr. Seddon suggests sleeping with your lenses out at least once or twice a week to be safe. "The results of our study suggest that your risk of ulceration increases 5 percent every night you sleep with extended-wear lenses in," she says.

Dr. Seddon and her colleagues found that the other major risk factor for ulcerative keratitis was lens hygiene—or, more specifically, the lack of it. "The overall level of lens care was alarmingly low" in everyone they studied, the doctors wrote. When you're cleaning your lenses, don't overlook the case you keep them in. "The lens case should be scrubbed clean with water every other day or so," Dr. Seddon says.

We shouldn't have to make this last point, but the medical researchers say we do: "There is one thing that all eye doctors agree no one should *ever* do, and that's put a lens in your mouth!"

—*Martha Capwell*

High-Tech Socks

Want to be blister free at last? Invest a few bucks in the latest style foot protection and you'll never blister again.

● ●

FOR SO MANY OF US, the thrill of working out is all too often muted by the agony of the feet. That's because when it comes to selecting athletic footgear, many men concentrate on shoes but overlook the socks. Yes, socks.

According to Wayne Axman, D.P.M., a New York triathlete who is also a sports podiatrist, men will spend hours poring over shoe guides, comparing information on the midsoles and cushioning properties of basketball, tennis, running and hiking shoes, and then plunk down a C note and some change for a high-tech model. But when it comes to socks, they go no-tech and rummage through their drawers for anything handy.

Guilty as charged. I used to be like that. I always mixed the latest in shoe technology with cheapo socks. Not only was my sock collection thin—as in socks worn and frayed in the heel and toe-box areas—but at times I even played full-court hoops sockless if I couldn't round up a pair at game time.

Times have changed and so have I. Instead of wearing the same socks for cycling, basketball and running, my particular sport passions, I now wear different types of socks for each. The sport-specific socks now found in athletic stores are more than just filler for your shoes, more than covering for the feet. They're integral pieces of sports equipment, just like your shoes. Materials such as polypropylene, Lycra, spandex, high-bulk acrylic, CoolMax and Thermax have been added to socks, almost eliminating natural fibers.

REAL COMFORT FROM SYNTHETICS

Some podiatrists say these new synthetic socks are better for you than the old standbys like cotton or wool. It all has to do with wicking, the ability of synthetics to effectively move perspiration from the foot. "Yes, cotton socks may initially feel comfortable when you put them on," says Rosario J. La Barbera, D.P.M., past president of the American Podiatric Medical Association, "but once you run a few miles in cotton socks or play a set of tennis in them, the sweat buildup remains with the fabric. And that's what leads to blisters, thickened toenails and fungal infections."

"Socks that are made of 100 percent acrylic or blends of natural and synthetic fibers are the way to go," agrees Douglas H. Richie, D.P.M., a Seal Beach, California, podiatrist whose sock tests at the Long Beach Marathon confirmed that runners in synthetic-based socks suffered fewer blisters than those wearing cotton socks.

Synthetic fibers also retain their shape and texture longer. After a few machine washings, cotton socks without the added resilient synthetics become limp and shapeless. Synthetics tend to bounce back to their original shape. One caution: Bleach can damage synthetic fibers. Wash as directed.

Beyond the new materials, the very construction of socks is different today. Basketball socks have a high heel cushion to minimize pressure from the sneaker heel. Tennis socks come with ribbed insteps to help dissipate lace pressure. Ski socks come with reinforced shin shields to protect against "boot bang." In addition, there are specialty socks made for mountain-bike riding, walking, fishing, hiking, snowboarding, golf, soccer and baseball, many of them with added shock absorption to protect your feet from the wear and tear of running. "When you run, each footfall brings down approximately two to three times your body weight on your foot," Dr. Axman says. "A good pair of athletic shoes, along with well-padded socks, will absorb a lot of that pounding."

Let's look at the advantages, sock by sock.

ALL-PURPOSE

Double Lay-R Cross Trail Fitness Sock ($7.95) has Kevlar (the same material used in bulletproof vests) added to the toes and heel for extra durability.

PrimaSport Crew ($5.75) offers a fully cushioned forefoot to minimize foot impact in running and jumping, and Bioguard, a special odor killer that's said to last the life of the socks.

Ridgeview CoolMax Cross-Trainer ($5.75) is lightweight and made with an exclusive channel fiber to wick perspiration away from the skin.

RUNNING

Nike CoolMax Run/Cycle Sock ($5.75) is a sleek, totally cushionless sock that fits like a glove and is recommended for those who want to feel the technical features of their shoes.

PrimaSport Wicking Quarter Top ($6.25) is a synthetic blend designed to keep your feet dry.

Ridgeview CoolMax Running Sock ($4.50) is excellent for perspiration control. The synthetic CoolMax fiber is superior for wicking sweat away.

Thor-Lo JMX Mini-Crew ($7.50) features an extra-thick, spongy impact zone at the ball and heel, with lower-density padding at the arch so the sock doesn't bunch up.

Thor-Lo RMX ($6.50) is a midweight designed for racers that offers even more shock absorption, while the stretch nylon instep provides a "sockless" feel.

BIKING

Brilliant CoolMax model ($4.50) will keep your feet cool and dry, and the colors will make you hard to miss.

Double Lay-R ATB 54 ($6.95) is designed for the serious mountain-bike rider. Both toe and heel are reinforced with Kevlar for durability. The sock has a black cuff so dirt stains won't be a problem.

Performance Pro Line socks ($5.95) combine high-wicking CoolMax fiber and special vented side panels for improved breathability.

● ●

Loose Shoes

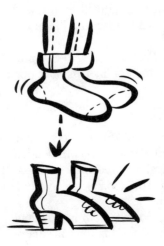

Wearing the wrong shoe causes most foot problems, according to the American Health Foundation. So take charge of your shoe shopping with these tips.

■ **Always have your feet measured: They may have changed from exercise or weight loss.**
■ **Put your full weight on the foot as it's measured.**
■ **Everybody has one foot that's larger: Use the bigger one to determine your size.**
■ **Wait at least until noon to make sure your feet have expanded to their true size.**
■ **Leave ½ inch between your toe and the tip of the shoe.**
■ **Make sure the shoe bends where your foot does.**
■ **Don't figure on breaking in uncomfortable shoes.**

PrimaSport CoolMax Quarter Top ($6.50) uses CoolMax for perspiration control and a Spandex top to keep the socks from rolling down.

Thor-Lo CMC ($7) is an ultrathin sock that's padded in the heel and ball for shock absorption and has CoolMax to draw off the sweat.

RACQUET SPORTS

Nike Court Crew ($7) blends CoolMax with cotton to offer a sock that protects against friction during lateral court movement.

PrimaSport Court CoolMax Quarter Top ($5.75) offers what they call a Landing Pad cushioning system, which uses ribbing in the sole and toe for shock absorption and to prevent foot slide.

Ridgeview Tennis Sock ($4.75) features Duraspun, a synthetic fiber that provides bulk and cushioning for maximum shock absorption, along with good perspiration-wicking.

Thor-Lo Tennis Crew TX ($8) blends acrylic and nylon fibers and is thickly padded at the ball and heel, with a pad over the toe to protect against skin abrasion.

BASKETBALL

PrimaSport Over the Calf ($7) offers special calf support.

Ridgeview Basketball Sock ($5.25), used by many NBA players, offers high-bulk Duraspun fiber for extra shock absorption.

Thor-Lo BX Basketball Sock ($8) features an extended heel pad to protect the Achilles tendon.

HIKING

Double Lay-R Lightweight Field Combo Pak ($17.95) actually consists of two different socks, a CoolMax boot liner to wick moisture away from the foot and an outer sock of poylpropylene, nylon and wool that you wear over the liner. It is guaranteed to keep your feet blister free.

PrimaSport Thermax Over The Calf ($12.50) combines Thermax and wool for superior warmth during cool- and cold-weather hiking, fishing and mountaineering.

Thor-Lo KX Hiking Crew Sock ($8.50) is padded in the heel and the ball of the foot to protect against blisters and abrasion. Use for day trips or easy overnights when you're not carrying too much weight.

—Gerald Couzens

Part 9

BOD LIKE
A ROCK

It's Supposed to Be
Fun, Right?

*Here are myths about exercise you wish
somebody had debunked when you
were in junior high gym class.*

••••••••••••••••••••••

WHEN IT COMES TO myths, there may be more about
exercise than just about anything. Here are 15 you've probably
heard at one time or another.

1. It's supposed to be fun. Sometimes it is, sometimes
it isn't. Fun really isn't the point. The point is how good you
feel *after* you've put your body through its paces.

2. Sit-ups flatten your belly. They'll tone your stomach muscles, but they won't do much to any fat that covers those muscles. You can't spot reduce with exercise; if you could, people who chew gum a lot would all have thin faces.

3. You'll lose weight. The scale is not a good measure of how well your exercise program is working. If you lift weights, for example, you'll lose flab; but because you're losing fat tissue and replacing it with denser, heavier muscle tissue, your weight may stay the same. The important thing is, you'll look better.

4. You should work out before you eat. Only partly true. If you're more than 30 percent above your ideal weight, exercising before a meal will burn up more calories. If you're less than 30 percent overweight, exercising *after* eating burns more calories. (To avoid indigestion, however, you probably won't want to do any serious aerobic exercise too soon after eating a heavy meal.)

5. Machines are better than free weights. Machines may be more convenient, even safer in some cases, but you can build just as much muscle if you learn how to use barbells and dumbbells.

6. Weight lifters should eat extra protein. Most of us already have too much protein in our diets. Although exercising will use up some protein, your current intake is probably more than adequate to replenish it.

7. Morning is the best time to exercise. There's no evidence that exercising at a particular time of day is significantly more beneficial. The best time to exercise is when you most feel like exercising. If you're not a morning person, you're not going to stick with an a.m. workout program for long. The only caveat is that exercising too close to bedtime may make it more difficult for you to fall asleep.

8. Stretching afterward can help prevent muscle pain. Studies show that stretching after a workout has no effect on muscle soreness.

9. You have to do it for 30 continuous minutes to get any benefit. A study at Stanford University showed that 10 minutes of exercise three times a day is almost as good. In any case, a little exercise every day, even if it's just a walk, is a lot better than none at all.

10. When you stop, muscle turns to fat. Hard muscles may turn into soft muscles, but they won't turn into fat. Muscle cells and fat cells are completely different, and neither can ever turn into the other.

11. Sooner or later, you'll get hurt. Injuries are far from inevitable. In fact, the majority of exercisers don't get hurt. Of those that do, the most common cause is overuse. The best way to avoid injuries is to increase the intensity and duration of your exercise a little at a time.

12. After a good sweat, you'll need extra salt. You'd have to shed three quarts of sweat to lose just *half* of the 9 to 12 grams of salt the average man consumes in a day. Since it's highly unlikely you'll sweat anything close to that amount, there's no reason to add extra salt to your diet or to take salt pills after hot-weather workouts.

13. Sit-ups are best done with hands behind your neck. Not if you don't want to wreck that neck. Doing sit-ups with your hands behind your neck puts too much pressure on cervical vertebrae. Keep your hands on your chest.

14. People with high blood pressure shouldn't lift weights. People with high blood pressure, or any cardiovascular problem, should see their doctors before undertaking a strength-training exercise program, but long-term effects of weight lifting on blood pressure have failed to show any negative effects, and some have demonstrated that the exercises can *reduce* blood pressure.

15. No pain, no gain. Ignore pain, no brain. You can get very fit without feeling any serious discomfort, so don't strain when you train. If it hurts, stop it.

—Michael Lafavore

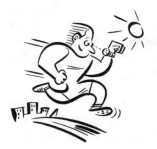

Matinee Magic
You can generally get a more intense workout when you exercise in the afternoon because the body's strength and aerobic capacities are slightly greater then, says a report in *The Physician and Sportsmedicine.*

No-Pain Gain

*Straight from the American College
of Sports Medicine, here's a sport-by-sport
guide to injury-free training.*

●●●●●●●●●●●●●●●●●●●●●

WHEN WE WERE KIDS, we didn't have to worry much about sports injuries. Our bodies seemed to be made from some indestructible material. We could run for miles, ride our bikes until the chains fell off and throw ourselves around on a baseball diamond hour after hour without suffering so much as a sore muscle. If, by some mishap, we did get hurt, we healed so quickly that it hardly mattered.

At a certain age—around the far turn of 25 or so—things started to change. Those grand impulses to slide into the cleats of the second baseman in the annual Little League father-son game got us into more trouble than they were worth. A too-long weekend run could make us hobble for a week. Just putting a little extra snap into the tennis swing or golf stroke became capable of sidelining us with back or shoulder problems.

Still, it would be a big mistake to use our body's greater susceptibility to injury as an excuse to become mere spectators. The benefits of an active lifestyle still far outweigh the potential risk of injury. It's just that we've got to be willing to acknowledge that the old bones and joints and muscles aren't quite as invulnerable as they once seemed.

To help you enjoy sports without enduring the bangs, bruises, bashes, twists and strains, *Men's Health* teamed up with selected members of the world's leading organization in sports medicine and exercise science, the American College of Sports Medicine. After spending time with some of the college's 12,000 physicians, exercise physiologists, physical therapists, nutritionists, trainers and coaches, we compiled this guide to injury-free training.

RUNNING

Running probably exacts more of a toll on the body than any other sport. With each stride, the runner's body absorbs a force equal to two to three times his own body weight. This hammers muscles, joints and tendons. Although advances in shoe technology have helped protect them from some of the pounding, runners typically lose more training time to injuries than any other athletes.

Most common injuries: Hamstring pulls, Achilles tendinitis, shin splints (inflammation of the soft tissue in the lower leg), stress fractures in feet or lower leg.

Number of injuries treated in hospital per year: 59,525.

Injury-Free Training Tips

1. Walk as well as run. Especially when starting a running program, it's smart to blend in some walking. It's easier on the joints, muscles and tendons, and mile for mile, it burns almost the same number of calories as running, says cardiologist Paul Thompson, M.D., a former 2:28 marathoner.

2. Balance your body. Running primarily strengthens the muscles in the *back* of the legs (the calves and hamstrings) while neglecting the quadriceps in the front. To balance out any strength differences, runners should do exercises such as squats and leg extensions to build up their quadriceps. Also, runners should stretch before and after running to keep calves and hamstrings as flexible and shock-absorbent as possible.

3. Run in running shoes; walk in walking shoes. "Many runners live in their running shoes, and this is asking for injury," says Dr. Thompson. Running shoes have very little heel, and they tend to leave the Achilles tendon unsupported when you walk. Walking shoes don't offer enough cushioning for a run.

4. Up your mileage gradually. Trying to do too much too soon is probably the surest way to get hurt. A good rule of thumb is never to increase your weekly mileage by more than 10 percent.

5. Run on soft surfaces. Choose dirt or grass-covered trails over concrete or asphalt.

SWIMMING

More Americans participate in swimming than any other sport, and that makes doctors very happy. Unlike dry-land athletes, swimmers don't have to support their own weight, so their bodies are spared the jarring forces that so often cause injuries. When swimmers do hurt themselves, the injuries are usually from overuse or improper form.

Most common injuries: Swimmer's shoulder (rotator-cuff strains or tears), elbow tendinitis, knee pain.

Number of injuries treated in hospital per year: 33,407.

Injury-Free Training Tips

1. Get your strokes down. Improper stroke techniques are the cause of many swimming injuries, says Rick Sharp, Ph.D., editor of the *Journal of Swimming Research.* Have a knowledgeable swimmer or coach analyze your stroke to correct any mechanical problems.

2. Mix it up. Doing a variety of strokes during your swim workout will decrease your chances of suffering an overuse injury.

3. Keep things rolling. Shoulder injuries are more common in freestyle swimmers who have a flat stroke than in those who roll their shoulders into the water.

4. Turn up the volume slowly. Like other endurance athletes, swimmers tend to get injured when they try to do too much too soon. Never increase the amount of swimming you do in a single workout or training week by more than 10 percent.

RACQUETBALL

Locked in a small room with one or more racket-swinging opponents and a hard rubber ball cruising at 80 to 100 miles an hour, racquetball players are at considerable risk for eye injury. But also common are lacerations and bruises from head-on collisions with walls and opponents, muscle pulls and strains from overly vigorous serves and returns, and joint and ligament sprains and tears from the constant stop-start action.

Most common injuries: Elbow and wrist tendinitis, ankle sprains, hamstring pulls, eye injuries, lacerations.

Number of injuries treated in hospital per year: 12,944.

Injury-Free Training Tips

1. Learn your strokes. As with any racket sport, improper stroke mechanics are the surest path to overuse injuries like elbow or wrist tendinitis, says Garron Weiker, M.D., administrative director of the Section of Sports Medicine at the Cleveland Clinic Foundation. Even if you've been playing for several years, sign up for a session with a teaching pro who can evaluate your strokes and tell you if you need to make any changes.

2. Get a good racket. A high-quality racket with a comfortable grip can help reduce tendinitis-producing vibration and shock. (Whether you choose aluminum or graphite makes little difference from an injury standpoint as long as the racket is well made, notes Dr. Weiker.)

3. Watch your eyes. Eye protection is a must for all racquetball players. "Although many players wear open [i.e., lensless] goggles, these do not give full protection since a speeding racquetball can bulge through the opening," says Dr. Weiker. Wraparound goggles with solid polycarbonate lenses are your best bet.

4. Get court shoes. Rubber-soled racquetball shoes are the best for the game, but in a pinch, a tennis, basketball or cross-training shoe will give you the heel support and cushioning you need to avoid injury.

TENNIS

Nearly half of all tennis players suffer from tennis elbow (pain usually caused by tendinitis) at least once. The problem stems from repeatedly making strokes that require wrist action and rotation of the forearm. Tennis players also suffer from lower back and shoulder injuries resulting from vigorous serves and overheads. Tears and sprains in the leg muscles are also common because of the stop-start motion required for the game.

Most common injuries: Shoulder and elbow tendinitis, knee tendinitis and cartilage damage, back strains, rotator-cuff tears.

Number of injuries treated in hospital per year: 34,674.

Injury-Free Training Tips

1. Muscle up. Contrary to common belief, frequent tennis playing actually *weakens* the shoulder muscles by stretching and fatiguing the tissues there, says Robert Nirschl, M.D., medical director and orthopedic consultant at the Virginia Sports Medicine Institute in Arlington. To reduce their risk of shoulder injury, tennis players need to perform strengthening exercises targeting the arms and shoulders. Good exercises include wrist curls, shoulder shrugs and shoulder rolls.

2. Get good form. "Improper technique can cause a whole host of injuries," says Dr. Nirschl. Even if you've been playing for years, the odds are that your stroke mechanics could use some fine-tuning. Taking a lesson or two every month will help you develop and maintain proper form.

3. Stretch your back before you play. For a simple stretch, lie on your back, grasp one leg underneath the knee with both hands and gently pull it toward your chest, then repeat with the other leg.

4. Go graphite. Graphite rackets are lightweight and strong, a perfect combination for damping injury-producing vibration.

5. Don't be so tense. String the racket at the lowest tension possible. High string tensions provide good control over the ball but pass along more vibration to the arm.

6. Get tennis shoes. Tennis shoes are specifically designed to give you the right traction, cushioning and heel support to keep your feet and lower legs healthy after hours on the court. In a pinch, cross-training shoes will do the trick, although by using them you may sacrifice some traction and support.

BASKETBALL/VOLLEYBALL

With all their quick starts, sudden stops and sky-high leaps, these two sports are among the most exciting around. But all this excitement does have its price, especially for the unprepared body. First, there's the tremendous amount of lateral force both place on ankles and knees. Then there's the bone- and joint-jarring jumping, which sends injurious shock waves throughout the body. All this adds up to a simple, undeniable conclusion: Basketball and volleyball players who want to stay healthy need to work extra hard between games to stay in shape.

Most common injuries: Ankle sprains, knee cartilage or ligament strains and tears, knee or Achilles tendinitis, assorted muscle strains.

Number of injuries treated in hospital per year: basketball, 465,616; volleyball, 87,023.

Injury-Free Training Tips

1. Get the right shoes. Shoes designed specifically for basketball or volleyball provide the support, cushioning and traction needed to play the game injury free, says Bert Mandelbaum, M.D., team physician at Pepperdine University in California. Wear high tops, especially if you have weak ankles. Doing so can greatly reduce the chance of reinjuring a previously sprained or strained ankle.

2. Prepare your body. The constant jumping and stop-start motion of basketball and volleyball can easily injure muscles that aren't trained to deal with these motions. Agility drills (doing short bursts of running from side to side) can help prepare an athlete's body to absorb these tremendous forces, says Peter Bruno, M.D., internist for the New York Rangers and Knicks.

3. Protect your eyes for basketball. Though it's not officially a contact sport, elbows and hands do tend to find their way into your eyes. To best protect your visual assets without reducing your vision, use wraparound polycarbonate lenses. The lenses are lightweight and unbreakable, and they provide protection from all possible angles.

4. Get padded for volleyball. If you're one of those players who'll do anything to put themselves between the ball and the floor, wear neoprene elbow pads and kneepads.

BASEBALL

Anyone who repeatedly throws a ball at high speeds is at risk of damaging his rotator cuff, the group of muscles and tendons that surround the shoulder joint. To protect this sensitive area, it's essential to work on upper-body strength and flexibility. And since baseball itself does little to improve overall fitness, it is extremely important for baseball players to maintain their own independent conditioning program.

Most common injuries: Elbow or shoulder tendinitis, rotator-cuff tears, bruises and scrapes.

Number of injuries treated in hospital per year: 280,652.

Injury-Free Training Tips

1. Build gradually. Throwing too much or too hard at the beginning of the season is a sure way to injure untrained muscles, says Dennis Wilson, Ed.D., head of the Department of Health and Human Performance at Auburn University in Alabama.

2. Muscle up. Although it's impossible to *strengthen* the rotator cuff itself with a single exercise, you can protect it by doing weight-lifting exercises to build the shoulder and upper back muscles. Lateral raises, rowing-type exercises and lat pulldowns are all great exercises for baseball players.

3. Warm up. Although baseball requires explosive bursts of activity, the game itself provides little opportunity for a player to warm his muscles. Thus it's necessary to make time for a pregame warm-up consisting of some short jogs and stretches for the shoulders, back and legs.

4. Get spiked. Molded-plastic cleats are best for baseball since they provide more traction than running or court shoes and they're less dangerous than metal spikes.

CYCLING

Even though cycling doesn't involve the pounding common to many sports, bike riders suffer more injuries than any other group of athletes. Falls do most of the damage, but the constant pedaling can also cause injury by repeatedly stressing the same muscles. Finally, the prolonged hunched-over position puts cyclists at risk for back pain.

Most common injuries: Knee tendinitis, low back strains, cuts and scrapes.

Number of injuries treated in hospital per year: 580,119.

Injury-Free Training Tips

1. Put a lid on. The majority of cycling injuries are the result of crashes or falls. A recent study found that one life could be saved every day in the United States if all cyclists were to wear helmets.

2. Get a good fit. Many cyclists experience chronic back and knee pain from improper positioning on their bikes, says Jim Hagberg, Ph.D., exercise physiologist at the University of Maryland. To get a proper fit, have an experienced rider or bike mechanic check the position of your saddle, handlebars and cleats.

3. Train your stomach. Building strong abdominal muscles can give your back the support it needs while you're cycling. Do abdominal strengthening exercises like crunches two or three times a week to ward off back pain.

4. Spin, don't strain. Although using bigger, higher gears can make you go faster, it can also make you more susceptible to muscle strains and other overuse injuries. "Using lower gears and a faster pedal stroke is not only easier on the body, it's also more efficient," says Dr. Hagberg.

5. Wear proper cycling shoes. Firm-soled cycling shoes make pedaling more efficient and help reduce strain on your feet.

6. Protect your eyes. Sunglasses not only reduce fatigue from the sun's glare but also keep flying debris and insects out of your eyes. When shopping for glasses, look for ones with polycarbonate lenses that are labeled "special purpose." The polycarbonate material prevents shattering, while the special-purpose label ensures maximum protection from the sun's ultraviolet rays.

BOWLING

Once-a-week bowlers run the risk of straining underdeveloped muscles from hefting those 16-pound balls. And those who bowl daily are at risk for overuse injuries. Whether you're an avid bowler or gutter-ball specialist, it pays to prepare for the demands the sport places on your body.

Most common injuries: Elbow tendinitis, wrist tendinitis, knee, back and shoulder strains, blisters.

Number of injuries treated in hospital per year: 22,515.

Injury-Free Training Tips

1. Watch that hook. Trying to put too much spin on the ball is one of the major causes of bowling injuries. If you decide you need to develop a spin delivery, switch to a lighter ball until you get the form down.

2. Adjust your form to your physique. If you have a bad back, don't bend at the back as much when you throw; instead, bend your knees to get low to the ground for your delivery. If you've had a knee injury, bend more at the back and keep your knees a bit straighter for your delivery.

3. Don't whip it. A smooth delivery that allows you to put your entire body behind the ball is the most effective, and safest, way to generate ball speed. Whipping or jerking the ball from your shoulder greatly increases your risk of injury—and gutter balls.

4. Don't rent shoes. Even if you only bowl once a month, it's both fiscally and physically wise to buy your own shoes. Not only will they look better, they'll also give you the proper fit and traction you need to ward off injuries.

GOLF

Golfers are susceptible to back injuries. With every swing of the club, a golfer bends forward, rotates at the hips and then follows through with as much force and speed as he can muster. All this puts tremendous strain on both the lower and upper back muscles.

Most common injuries: Low back strains, shoulder strains, shoulder, wrist and elbow tendinitis.

Number of injuries treated in hospital per year: 35,218.

Injury-Free Training Tips

1. Stay loose. Since golf involves a great deal of rotation at the shoulders and hips, keeping these areas flexible is the most important thing golfers can do to prevent injuries, says Lewis Yocum, M.D., assistant medical director for the Professional

Golfers' Association of America. For a simple shoulder stretch, raise your right arm straight above your head, then bend it at the elbow so your right hand falls behind your neck. With your left hand, gently pull your right elbow. Stop when you feel a gentle stretch in your right shoulder and hold for five seconds. Repeat with the other arm. To stretch your back and hips, stand with your feet flat on the floor, shoulder-width apart. While holding a golf club behind your neck, twist your upper body gently from side to side without moving your feet.

2. Muscle up. Strengthening your back and abdominal muscles will also decrease your chance of golf injuries. The best exercises for golf involve rotational motion. Try diagonal sit-ups (where you alternately bring your right elbow to your left knee and left elbow to your right knee).

3. Use the proper shoes. As in any other sport, having the right shoes for golf is vital. You really do need those little spikes to hold your feet in place as you make the backswing. As for the tassels, well, it's your call.

4. Take a lesson. Improper form greatly increases your risk of injury. To keep yourself from developing any bad habits

• •

Steer Clear of Steer before a Workout

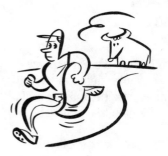

Steer clear of protein-rich foods like beef just before a heavy workout. They may make exercise tougher. In one study, athletes who loaded up on protein an hour before a treadmill run felt they had to work harder at their workouts than did peers who had only water beforehand. Researchers speculate that protein diverts oxygen to digestion—and away from working muscles—more than other nutrients do. A better pre-warm-up snack: a couple of fig bars, a banana or an energy bar.

in your game, take a few lessons from a teaching pro at your local golf course. Even if you have a five handicap, it's a good idea to have a pro analyze your stroke at least once a season.

5. Don't whack it. A fluid stroke that generates a lot of club speed is the key to driving a golf ball far down the fairway. "Trying to muscle a ball off the tee will only get you injured," says Dr. Yocum. Also, when practicing your drive, hit off a soft surface like grass. Constantly hitting off a hard plastic mat transfers a great deal of shock to your lower arm and can cause tendinitis.

6. Squat, don't bend. There's a lot of reaching to place or pick up balls in this game. Bending over at the waist can put a great deal of strain on your lower back. Remember to bend your knees before leaning forward.

(For further information on fitness and sports medicine, contact the American College of Sports Medicine at 317-637-9200.)

—Dan Bensimhon

Damage Control

*Ooow! Sometimes, despite all precautions,
sports injuries happen. Here's what
to do when you're hurting.*

•••••••••••••••••••••••

PLAYING SPORTS IS SUPPOSED to be fun. It's not supposed to hurt. If it's more pain than pleasure, you're definitely doing something wrong. Usually such twinges, strains, muscle pulls and cramps are your body's way of telling you that you've been pushing too hard. Pay attention.

Probably the most common of all exercise pains is *muscle soreness,* dull pain that usually shows up within a day of strenuous exercise. There's no reason to stop exercising because of a minor ache, but go easy for a day or two. Gentle stretching

• •

R.I.C.E. TO THE RESCUE

When it comes to treating injuries like sprains, pulls and tears, R.I.C.E. is the gold standard among sports-medicine professionals. This treatment helps to reduce the damage and swelling caused by an injury and can significantly speed healing.

Rest. Stop exercising—immediately. Decrease weight on the injured area (or eliminate it altogether) to prevent any further damage.

Ice. Apply ice wrapped in a towel or plastic bag to the injured spot for 10 to 20 minutes three to four times a day until acute injury subsides.

Compress. Apply pressure to the area by wrapping it in a snug (but not tight) elastic bandage.

Elevate. Lift the injured limb 12 to 18 inches and rest it on a pillow or cushion. This will reduce swelling.

• •

and a massage can also help reduce the stiffness associated with muscle aches. The ache should disappear completely within 72 hours. If it doesn't, see a doctor.

Muscle cramps can range from a mildly painful lockup of a muscle group to an agonizing stabbing feeling. What's happening is a lot like what it *feels* is happening: Your muscle has contracted and won't release. It's usually caused by muscle fatigue, dehydration or chemical imbalance. If you get a cramp while exercising, stop or slow down until the pain goes away. (It usually will in a minute or two.) Some find that stretching or rubbing the muscle helps speed the recovery process.

Muscle strains and pulls range from mild overstretching to an actual tear. Sometimes the first signal is a twinge during a workout; other times the pain is sudden and searing. In the first case, go easy and see if the pain dissipates. If not, or if the pain is severe, stop exercising and treat the injury with R.I.C.E. (see "R.I.C.E to the Rescue" above). Consult a doctor if pain hasn't begun to ease within 48 hours. A strain may take several weeks to heal.

Here, from the American College of Sports Medicine, are some more specific tips on dealing with sports injuries.

FOOT

Symptoms: Sharp pain directly over one of the bones in the foot, usually accompanied by slight swelling. Pain increases during exercise or when standing for long periods.

Probable injury: Stress fracture of one of the small bones in the foot, often caused by the repetitive pounding of running.

Treatment: Stop activity. See a physician.

Prevention: Wear shoes with good cushioning. Run on softer surfaces such as grass or an indoor track. Increase training gradually.

Symptoms: Pain and tenderness that begin in the heel and radiate into the midsection of the foot. Pain lessens during activity but returns intensely an hour or so after stopping.

Probable injury: Plantar fasciitis, an inflammation of the connective tissue that runs from the heel bone to the base of the toes and supports the bottom of the foot.

Treatment: Rest. Ice. Over-the-counter pain relievers (before taking any medication, check with your physician on dosage, indications and side effects). Orthotics to reduce overpronation and remove stress from the fascia.

Prevention: Wear shoes with good arch support and cushioning. Use orthotics to prevent overpronation. Keep fascia flexible and strong by scrunching up a towel with your toes.

ANKLE

Symptoms: Pain and swelling, usually on outside of ankle after trauma. Commonly accompanied by bruising.

Probable injury: Ankle sprain, a stretching or tearing of the ankle ligaments. Damage ranges from mild overstretching to complete rupture.

Treatment: R.I.C.E. If pain persists or worsens over 48 hours, see a doctor.

Prevention: Keep ankles flexible and strong with the following exercise: Wrap a towel around the ball of your foot, and extend your ankle as you pull back on the towel to provide resistance. Wear a brace or high-top sneakers to support previously injured ankles. Run on even surfaces.

LOWER LEG

Symptoms: Burning pain on the back of the leg near the heel. Pain lessens with activity but returns soon after stopping. May be accompanied by swelling and redness.

Probable injury: Achilles tendinitis, an inflammation in the tendon that connects the calf muscle to the heel bone.

Treatment: Rest. Ice. Over-the-counter pain relievers. Stretch tendon gently when pain is gone by standing 18 inches from a wall and leaning into the wall while keeping feet flat on the floor. Place heel lift in shoe to decrease stretch of Achilles and help prevent reinjury.

Prevention: Wear shoes with adequate heel support and cushioning. Stretch regularly. Increase training gradually.

Symptoms: Sharp pain in the front or back of the lower leg that typically lessens with activity but returns intensely soon after stopping. In some cases, pain may be severe during exercise as well.

Probable injury: Shin splints, an inflammation of the soft tissues in the lower leg.

Treatment: Rest. Ice. Over-the-counter pain relievers.

Prevention: Strengthen lower leg by performing exercises such as heel raises and toe raises. Increase flexibility with calf stretches. Wear shoes with good cushioning. Increase training gradually. Run on soft surfaces.

KNEE

Symptoms: Deep ache or pain underneath the knee. Discomfort increases during activity, when bending or straightening knee, or when direct pressure is applied. May swell or grind.

Probable injury: Chondromalacia patellae ("runner's knee"), a wearing away of the back side of the kneecap and the cartilage that cushions it.

Treatment: Rest until pain subsides (may take several weeks). Over-the-counter pain relievers. If pain persists or grinding is present, see a doctor.

Prevention: Strengthen quadriceps to better support the knee by doing leg extensions. Stretch quadriceps and hamstrings. Wear well-cushioned shoes. Have running stride analyzed to correct biomechanical flaws.

Symptoms: Intense pain along joint line that intensifies with activity. Can be accompanied by swelling or locking of joint.

Probable injury: Strain or tear of knee cartilage or ligament.

Treatment: R.I.C.E. Over-the-counter pain relievers. If pain or swelling is very severe or persists for more than 72 hours, see a doctor.

Prevention: Some injury due to trauma may be unavoidable, but you can reduce risk. Strengthen quadriceps. Keep knee flexible with stretching exercises. Wear an elastic knee brace if you have prior knee injury.

UPPER LEG

Symptoms: Sharp pain on back of leg above knee can radiate to buttocks. Typically intensifies with exercise.

Probable injury: Strain or tear in the hamstring muscle or the tendons that run along the back of the upper leg. (Also possible back injury. See "Back" on the opposite page.)

Treatment: Rest. Ice. Switch to heat afterward, but only if it reduces pain more effectively. Gentle stretching when pain subsides. A good stretch: Lie on your back with your legs up against a wall. Slowly slide buttocks toward the wall until you feel a gentle tug at the back of your legs.

Prevention: Always warm up and stretch hamstrings before exercising. Strengthen hamstring muscles and quadriceps to remove any strength imbalances. Good hamstring exercise: leg curl on an exercise machine.

GROIN

Symptoms: Sharp pain in groin area that may radiate to upper thigh or lower abdomen. Typically intensifies with exercise or stretching.

Probable injury: Groin pull, a strain or partial tear in the muscles or tendons in the upper leg and lower abdomen.

Treatment: Rest. Ice. Switch to heat after first 24 hours if it helps relieve pain. Resume training gradually, as complete recovery may take up to several weeks.

Prevention: Warm up before doing any sprinting or vigorous exercise. Keep the muscles of the upper inner thighs strong and flexible. At-home method: Wearing light ankle weights, lie on your side, lift one leg and return slowly. Do ten repetitions. Repeat with other leg.

BACK

Symptoms: Ache or pain in lower back that typically subsides during exercise but can return with a vengeance afterward. Usually accompanied by stiffness. In severe cases it is difficult to sit or stand.

Probable injury: Strain in the lower back muscles. Possible herniated disk.

Treatment: Rest. Ice. Switch to heat afterward if it reduces pain better. Gentle stretching when pain subsides. See a doctor if pain intensifies over several days, radiates to buttocks or legs, or causes numbness or tingling.

Prevention: Increase flexibility of back muscles by stretching daily. Strengthen abdominal muscles to support the spine. Try stomach crunches: Lie on your back with knees bent, and curl your chin to your chest so your shoulders come a couple of inches off the ground. Always avoid quick, twisting motions or heavy lifting.

SHOULDER

Symptoms: Dull ache or pain typically felt in the outer part of the shoulder that may radiate into the upper arm. Pain usually becomes worse with exercise. May be accompanied by swelling or redness.

Probable injury: Tendinitis (inflammation of the shoulder tendons) or bursitis (inflammation of the tiny shock-absorbing sacs inside the shoulder joint).

Treatment: Rest. Ice. Over-the-counter pain relievers. Gentle stretching when pain subsides. For a shoulder stretch, grab your right elbow with your left hand and gently pull it across your chest. Repeat with other arm.

Prevention: Strengthen shoulder muscles with rowing exercises. Increase shoulder flexibility through stretching. Always warm up before vigorous exercise.

ELBOW

Symptoms: Sharp pain on outside of elbow that may radiate down forearm. Pain usually intensifies with exercise.

Probable injury: Tennis elbow, tendinitis in the elbow and surrounding portion of forearm.

Treatment: Rest. Ice. Over-the-counter pain relievers. If you continue to play, use a splint or brace to restrict wrist movement.

Prevention: Learn proper technique for your sport. Use proper equipment for your size and ability. Strengthen and stretch forearm muscles with wrist curls.

—*Dan Bensimhon*

Time Bandit

*Is your schedule already crammed with
too much work? Here are some ideas on
how to fit fitness into your day.*

•••••••••••••••••••••••

RON HILL REMEMBERS the day as if the past 21 years had been but a blink: the time (not much), the place (a ramshackle train platform in Stuttgart, West Germany), the reason (a hurried trip to the 1969 European track championships in Budapest).

Five years earlier, after running poorly in the Tokyo Olympics, the Englishman had vowed never again to waver in his training. And he stuck to it; not a day passed without a run. Now, though, Hill's day was slipping away, the opportunity for laps with it. At Stuttgart, he did what had to be done. He hopped off the car and did a half mile near the station, capping his effort with a final sprint to catch the departing train.

"If you want to exercise you'll find the time. It's really no different than finding the time to shave or eat," reasons Hill, who currently fits two daily runs into a hectic schedule as owner of a sportswear business in Cheshire, England. "If you want to do it, you'll do it."

The benefits of exercise have been breathlessly documented by everyone from cardiologists to reformed rock stars, every newly minted expert urging us to walk, run, heft and gyrate. Unfortunately, this advice is often effectively smothered by a more pertinent question: Where's the time?

First, realize that a little effort goes a long way. "If all you want to do is enjoy a long, healthy life, it doesn't take that much activity at all," says Kenneth Cooper, M.D., head of the Dallas-based Institute for Aerobics Research. On the other hand, there's Dr. Cooper's coronary corollary: "The majority of the patients I take care of, the ones that don't have time for fitness," he says, "find the time after that first heart attack. Time is really just an excuse."

NO EXCUSES

Finding time, say experienced exercisers, is a matter of discipline and organization. Brent Knudsen, a 34-year-old triathlete and vice-president of marketing for a Fortune 500 company, trains every day, despite the demands of a 55-hour workweek. His regimen includes bicycling, running and a lunchtime swim at a health club.

What he does, though, isn't as important as how he does it. He maps out a schedule at the beginning of each month and then sticks to it as best he can. Planning a month in advance, Knudsen admits, is "probably a little extreme," but a schedule, even an elastic one, is essential to any successful exercise program.

"You have to schedule exercise into your day just like you'd schedule in a business meeting and, just like a business meeting, make it a priority," says Knudsen, who lives in La Jolla, California. "A lot of times work will pile up, and by noon I'll be thinking, 'I just can't swim today.'

"I simply have to tell myself that I'm going to go, that I'm going to discipline myself and do it. The key is to schedule it and then commit to it."

When to fit in exercise is a matter of personal preference and, at times, no small degree of innovation. California triathlete Mike Pigg once killed time on a boat trip by carting along a stationary bike, lashing it to the deck, mounting up and spinning away. (This is a guy who apparently believes idle legs are the devil's workout; Pigg will talk to you while standing on one leg. "Builds up your knee and ankle," he explains.)

BLOW OFF YOUR DAY

Less attention-grabbing, maybe a bit more productive, Knudsen cycles nightly on a stationary bike while reading reports he set aside during the day. Hill, who gets a daily run in before breakfast, recommends working out early, as fewer conflicts are apt to pop up at 6:00 A.M. Others swear by the regenerative boost of a noon sweat. Exercising later in the day can help you blow off steam from work.

"When I get to 4:00 in the afternoon, I've just about had it with this place," says Tom Ponte, 45, an administrator with Aetna Life and Casualty in Hartford, Connecticut. Lately, he's been getting in at 8:00 A.M. so he can leave an hour early and put in 20 minutes to an hour at the company's fitness center.

The point is that *when* you choose to exercise is not as important as settling into a routine. "Once you establish a pattern you're less likely to miss a workout," explains Ponte, who

• •

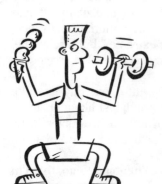

Too Thin? Work Out!

If you're too thin, don't pig out—work out. Weight training builds muscle bulk, says Rachel Barkley, assistant professor of clinical dietetics at the University of Oklahoma Health Sciences Center, but simply stuffing calories will puff you out without shaping you up. And like anyone else, skinny guys can wind up with high cholesterol problems from a high-fat diet.

has watched throngs of coworkers start a fitness program, miss a day or two, and then let everything fall by the wayside.

Fitness often seems like something you have to grab in big bunches. The truth is, in certain respects, exercise is really no different than sex or income-tax refunds. "A little bit is better than nothing," says Hill. "If all you have is 20 minutes to spare, get out there and use that 20 minutes. It's always worth the effort."

When it comes to finding time, a regular exercise program can have a beneficial backlash. "Generally, as people become more physically fit, they may find that they need less sleep," says Lisa Mueller, health promotion manager for Minneapolis-based Honeywell. "You may find yourself with more hours in the day to fit in exercise."

TRY PUSH-UPS

Whenever you're feeling time-crimped, Aetna exercise physiologist Doug Barber recommends one exercise above all others: push-ups. These gym-class stalwarts, combined with chair dips and crunches, make for a threesome that will work most of the major muscle groups of the upper body. Do 15 to 20 minutes of these strength exercises three times a week, along with about 20 minutes of cardiovascular work thrice weekly (walking, running, bicycling, etc.), and you'll get all the exercise you need, Barber says.

Other experts emphasize cross-training: choosing a number of exercises, then mixing them up as often as possible. This may seem straightforward, but a surprising number of people home in on one exercise, then butt heads with it until their brains turn to mush. As Doug Gambrel, an exercise physiologist for GTE Corporation in Stamford, Connecticut, says, "A variety of activities not only works muscles throughout the whole body but also keeps you fresh."

Variety, Gambrel points out, also allows for adaptability, especially important to the traveler trying to hack out an exercise program on unfamiliar, and sometimes unfriendly, turf. Running can take on a real sense of urgency in certain urban areas, but if you also lift weights or swim, it's easier to revise your schedule. Such revisions are made simpler still by the many hotels and handful of airports that offer in-house health facilities. Even if those facilities aren't available, there are still no excuses.

"If you make the commitment, you can get it done," says Tom Sullivan, a 42-year-old Hollywood actor, producer and lecturer who spent 220 days on the road last year and rarely missed a workout—an accomplishment all the more impressive considering he is blind.

Sullivan brings an elastic exercise band and a jump rope everywhere, but he actually starts each day by rolling out of bed and right to the floor for a short bout of calisthenics. It's a routine he has adopted out of respect for the realities of travel. "I don't care how disciplined you are, when you check into that hotel after a full day of traveling, exercise isn't at the top of your agenda. If you don't do it in the morning, you won't do it."

He also makes an attempt to eat lightly on the road, as does South African golf great Gary Player, who is a regimented exerciser. "Eating properly on the road is a great way to stay in shape," Player says. He makes a special effort to steer clear of fatty foods, no easy feat on the opulent Professional Golfers' Association tour.

MAKING TIME IS WORTH THE TIME

Let's face it, finding time for exercise can be a headache. And exercise itself is rarely the fuzzy buzz of orgiastic endorphins we would like it to be. So why not snap off the alarm and doze, forget the evening run and plow into the cheese dip?

That question is best answered by Walt Stack, who has rarely done either. As a laborer in San Francisco, Stack's day began at 2:40 in the morning, allowing him time to swim, bike and run before reporting to work at 7:30. Now that he is retired, his daily program, with minor alterations, consists of 14 miles of bicycling, 17 miles of running back and forth across the Golden Gate Bridge, and a quarter-mile swim in the bay.

Stack tells you what you probably already know.

"The difficult things in this world are solved through motivation," says Stack, who is 83. "No matter how tired you are, no matter how busy you are, if you're determined, you can always make the time. It's completely up to you."

—*Ken McAlpine*

Deflate Your Spare Tire

Lose your spare tire and you'll look better, feel better, have more energy and probably even live longer. Here are a dozen steps to a sleeker middle.

•••••••••••••••••••••••

THE SPARE TIRE SPARES no man. One day you wake up and you can no longer see the muscles in your abdomen. Your old pant size no longer fits comfortably in the waist. Shirts that used to look great on you are starting to spread a bit between the buttons.

Middle age has caught up with your middle section. Your genes, hormones and slowing metabolism are ganging up on your gut.

It's a simple fact that if you take in more calories than you burn, the extra get stored as fat. In men, more of that fat collects underneath the abdominal muscles than in other places—which is why some men can have rock-hard stomachs but still be thick at the equator.

Starting at about age 20, age-related changes begin to make it progressively easier for your belly to bulge. Most muscles and organs become smaller, and the body starts needing fewer calories to keep itself going. At the same time, your metabolism, or the rate at which the body burns calories, slows down.

Granted, these changes occur gradually. According to Jo-Ann Heslin, a registered dietitian and coauthor of *The Fat Attack Plan,* a man's metabolism slows only about 2 percent per decade after age 20.

"The catch is that while calorie requirements and metabolism are decreasing, most men are eating the same or more, and becoming less active," says Robert Kushner, M.D., director of the Nutrition and Weight Control Clinic at the University of Chicago. As a result, we stockpile calories. In the decade between ages 30 and 40 alone, the average man gains about six pounds.

All this is to say that a potbelly becomes more likely as you age. But it's not inevitable. The power to get rid of those extra inches is all yours. And there's good reason to do it. Lose your potbelly and you'll look better, feel better, have more energy and probably even live longer. Recent studies have linked potbellies with more serious problems such as heart disease, high blood pressure, stroke and diabetes.

Here, based on the latest research, are the best strategies for deflating that spare tire.

EXERCISE (BUT NOT NECESSARILY SIT-UPS)

Working out reverses the processes that cause a potbelly to form by revving up the metabolism and burning calories, explains Wayne Westcott, Ph.D., YMCA national strength-training consultant. Exercise helps you take pounds off and keep them off. In a long-term weight-loss study, men who exercised gained back only half the weight of men who just dieted. Here's what you need to know.

Aerobics target the belly. Recent research shows that when men burn fat with aerobic exercise, they lose it first and fastest in the abdomen.

In a study at the University of Washington in Seattle, men who took part in an intensive aerobic exercise program dropped 20 percent of the fat from their midsection in six months—almost twice the amount taken off arms and legs. Researchers dubbed this effect "preferential loss."

"Their shapes changed from round to more oblong," says researcher Robert S. Schwartz, M.D. "It was very obvious." He speculates that the more fat you have around the middle, the quicker you'll drop it with exercise.

Aerobic exercise is the cornerstone of any fat-burning plan because it does the most to fire up the metabolism. Any activity that boosts your heart rate above its resting pace for 30 minutes to an hour qualifies. Fat starts to melt away about 20 minutes into a workout, and the higher the heart rate, the more calories you'll burn. Aerobic exercise also makes your charged-up metabolism ignite calories even after you've quit your workout.

Top aerobic exercises for fat-burning include stair climbing, cross-country skiing, running and biking.

Lift weights to lose waist. Weight training, long maligned as an inefficient fat-burner, is now being hailed for its power to boost the benefits of aerobics. What's more, it speeds weight loss more than previously thought.

Weight training builds muscle, and muscle takes more energy to sustain itself than fat does. The more muscle you have, the higher your metabolism idles, not just after exercising, but *all* the time. "Every pound of muscle you add raises your daily calorie needs by 30 to 50 a day," says Dr. Westcott. "Over the course of an eight-week weight training program, if you gain three to five pounds of muscle—which is typical—you could be burning 250 extra calories a day just by sitting still."

This metabolic afterburn from weight training is one-third greater than that from aerobic exercise, according to a study at Oregon Health Sciences University.

The best results of all come with a one-two punch of weight training and aerobics. In a 16-week study at the University of Massachusetts, dieters doing both weights and aerobics lost more weight than dieters who did just one or the other.

Getting results from weights takes a surprisingly small commitment of time. Westcott recommends a 20-minute, thrice-weekly program requiring only one set on a typical circuit of either machines or free weights. This consists of about nine different exercises, each of which targets a major muscle group—biceps, triceps, upper back, lower back, pectorals, quadriceps, hamstrings, abdominals and shoulders. For each exercise, make the resistance heavy enough that muscles feel tired after 10 repetitions. When you can do 12 reps easily, increase the weight by 2½ to 5 pounds.

Isolate the abdominals. Can you target a bulging midsection with exercises like sit-ups and crunches? The prevailing evidence is that you cannot. Even if you were to do 300 sit-ups each and every day—and this has actually been tried in tests—you'd never work up enough aerobic steam to melt a single ounce of flab. But recent evidence shows that abdominal exercises do help in a different way. Sit-ups and crunches strengthen the muscles lying atop your inner fat cavity, and that can make your belly look smaller by altering your posture, says Ellington Darden, Ph.D., director of research for Nautilus Sports/Medical Industries and author of *32 Days to a 32-Inch Waist.*

According to Dr. Darden, a heavy abdomen can tug on the spine and cause it to arch forward. That sway in the back pushes the belly out further and can cause back strain to boot. Slow abdominal crunches help shore up the muscles that support the spine. "You're improving the whole girdle system of support in your midsection," he says.

He recommends one set of ten trunk curls and one set of ten reverse trunk curls. To do a trunk curl, lie on your back, with your arms crossed at the wrist above your chest, your knees bent and your feet flat on the floor. Slowly lift your shoulder blades, then your head, curling your chin toward your chest. Don't sit all the way up, but hold in a raised position for a count of five, then slowly lower your shoulders back to the floor. To do a reverse trunk curl, lie on your back and lift your hips toward the center of your chest. Keep your hands on the floor to help lift your buttocks off the mat.

EAT RIGHT

For most men, diets are the weapon of choice in the attack on fat. Unfortunately, diets don't usually work in the long term, especially if you lose weight quickly. "Some can even be harmful because they create mineral imbalances, loss of fluid, constipation and diarrhea," says Dr. Kushner. Is it any wonder they make some men depressed?

Still, what you take in has a direct bearing on what you store up (and where). The good news is that you don't necessarily have to cut back on how much you eat; it's what you eat that makes the difference. "Not all calories are equivalent. It matters where they come from," says Adam Drewnowski, Ph.D., director of the human nutrition program at the University of Michigan School of Public Health. Here's the best advice on eating right.

Cut fat. Studies show it's far more important to cut fat than calories. Eating fat will make you fat. "Fat is stored more easily and doesn't burn as fast as other nutrients," Dr. Kushner says. And in men, fat calories are most likely to be stored in the abdomen. (In women, fat goes mostly to the hips, thighs and buttocks.)

Researchers at Cornell University have made the astonishing finding that cutting fat intake can make you lose weight, *no matter how much food or how many calories you take in.* In one study, all subjects ate the same kind of food, but people in a low-fat group went without mayo on their turkey sandwiches, for example, or had low-fat instead of regular yogurt. Simple measures like this allowed them to cut fat to the 25 percent of calories that experts recommend we eat. (The average man gets about 38 percent of calories from fat.) After 11 weeks, the

• •

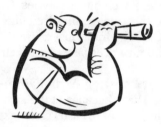

Finding a Healthy Health Club

Fitness guru Jack La Lanne and the Better Business Bureau have helpful hints for a first-class health club.

1. Try it before you buy it. Ask for a couple of day passes so you can use the club before you decide. "Question as many members as you can," advises La Lanne. "Ask them if they like the place and what they don't like about it."

2. Check for quality qualifications. Instructors should have bachelor's degrees in exercise physiology or similar fields, or certification by the American College of Sports Medicine.

3. Make sure the instructors instruct. It's essential that the instructors make sure the members are reaching their goals. "The instructors should get to know the members," says La Lanne.

4. Look up the report card. "There are so many fly-by-nights these days," says La Lanne. Ask for a reliability report from the local Better Business Bureau.

5. Read the fine print. Steer well clear of any club whose manager tries to make you sign a long-term contract right away. Ask if you can join on a month-to-month basis. If you are given a contract, take it home and read it over carefully.

low-fat eaters lost twice as much weight as people who ate more fat, even though there was no restriction on the total calories they consumed and the high-fat eaters limited calories to 2,000 per day.

The study's leader, David Levitsky, Ph.D., professor of nutrition and psychology, estimates that a low-fat diet can trim 10 percent off your body weight per year.

Easy ways to cut fat from your diet are to choose low-fat or nonfat milk, cheese and yogurt; eat lean cuts of meat and trim all visible fat; and fill up on vegetables, fruits and grain products like bread and pasta.

Load up on carbohydrates. Banish all notions that starches stick to the ribs. Carbohydrates burn fastest of all the body's energy sources and aren't easily converted into fat. When they are converted, the process itself burns calories. On top of that, carbohydrates spark the release of adrenaline, which burns still more calories. "Carbohydrates just cause the metabolic machinery in the body to turn over faster," says Dr. Kushner.

Weight-loss experts say that boosting carbohydrate intake will superheat a low-fat diet. That's because at the same time you're storing less fat by eating less of it, carbs can make your body work faster to burn the fat you have.

In one study, people placed on a fatty diet who tried to *maintain* the weight they had gained just couldn't do it when they switched to eating carbohydrates. What's more, most of the pounds they lost were fat. Body weight dropped about 3 percent on average, but body fat was cut by more than 11 percent.

Experts recommend you get about 60 percent of your calories from carbohydrates.

Tank up on water. Water's a secret weapon in the weight-loss war. Drinking more can help shed pounds in two ways.

First, it can take the edge off cravings. Often what seems like a craving for food is actually a craving for fluid, according to George L. Blackburn, M.D., Ph.D., chief of the Nutrition/Metabolism Laboratory at New England Deaconess Hospital in Boston. By drinking small sips of three or four ounces throughout the day—especially when you feel hungry—you can avert the need to indulge.

Second, if the water is ice cold, it can actually burn calories, according to Dr. Darden. "Ice-cold water is about 40°F," he says, "and it takes 226 calories of body heat to warm a gallon of it up to 98.6°." Dr. Darden recommends keeping an insulated 32-ounce bottle with a straw in it at your workplace all day. He advocates drinking four of these a day—double the usual recommendations for minimum daily fluid intake. But drinking that much icy water over a four-week period will make you drop about two pounds.

CUT DRINKING AND QUIT SMOKING

Experts say both alcohol and cigarettes cause changes in the body that make it easier for fat to pad the midsection. Here's the best advice.

Limit drinks to one a day (or thereabouts). That's what the Surgeon General recommends, and it sounds reasonable enough. But Michael Jensen, M.D., a consulting physician in nutrition, metabolism and internal medicine at the Mayo Clinic, knows this isn't how life works. One beer usually means three or four, at 100 to 200 calories per—"and that's just for the cheap stuff," he says. "That many beers, even if they're lights, could account for a third of your daily calories."

According to Dr. Jensen, there are three good reasons to cut back on alcohol if you want to lose a potbelly.

First, there are all those calories.

Second, since alcohol can't be stored the way other nutrients can, the body has to burn it off immediately. While the body's burning alcohol, it's *not* burning fat, which undermines the flab fight.

Third, beer isn't served with fruits and vegetables. "It's usually chips and dips and other things with a lot of fat and calories," Dr. Jensen says. "There's fat gain from circumstances."

One drink a day? "I wouldn't say you have to be so strict," Dr. Jensen concedes. "Make that an average. It's not the people who have an occasional three or four drinks that'll have a problem, but those who have three or four drinks *every day*."

Still, he adds, "if you're concerned about a potbelly, certainly alcohol is one of the first places to cut back."

If you smoke, stop. Some people argue that cigarettes keep you thin, since the average smoker weighs less than the average nonsmoker. But study after study shows that people who smoke—even if they're lighter than people who don't—tend to have bigger bellies. Scientists speculate that smoking causes hormones to steer more fat to the midriff. Quitting detours fat from the belly, so any weight that's gained tends to gather in the legs, resulting in a more balanced-looking shape, according to researcher Robert C. Klesges, Ph.D., associate professor of psychology at Memphis State University.

What's more, Dr. Klesges and others have found in studies that quitting brings lighter-than-normal smokers only up to the weight they would have been if they'd never smoked.

MAKING IT WORK

"To increase exercise and cut down on fat sounds simple enough, but it's really pretty tough because you have to work at it every day," says Carolyn Berdanier, Ph.D., a professor of nutrition at the University of Georgia. Here's what experts suggest to make your program a success.

Be a fat-tracker. To limit fat to 25 or 30 percent of your daily calories, you'll need to monitor your intake by reading labels.

To tell how many grams of fat are in a serving, lift the number straight from the label. Tally what you eat throughout the day. The average man takes in about 2,400 calories a day. To limit fat to 25 percent of that total, he should eat no more than 67 grams of fat per day.

For menu planning, paperback books like *The Fat Counter,* which Jo-Ann Heslin cowrote with another dietitian, Annette B. Natow, Ph.D., provide a handy fat tally for thousands of foods, including name-brand foods.

Set reasonable goals. To lose a pound of fat, you need to burn 3,500 more calories than you take in. That kind of combustion doesn't happen quickly. It's not realistic to figure on dropping 25 pounds in a month. How can you tell what *is* realistic? First, figure your target weight. To calculate that, give yourself 106 pounds for your first 5 feet of height. Add 6

●●

FAT GOALS

To limit fat to 25 percent of your total calorie intake, you should eat no more than the following amounts. (These figures apply to men only.)

Weight (lb.)	Calorie Intake	Fat Limit (g)
130	1,800	51
140	2,000	54
150	2,100	58
160	2,200	62
170	2,400	66
180	2,500	70
190	2,700	74
200	2,800	78

●●

pounds for each inch of height above that. For example, if you were 5-foot-9, you'd start with 106 pounds for the first 5 feet and add 54 (9 more inches times 6 pounds each). Your target weight would be 160. If you need to lose 20 pounds or less, you can reasonably do it in two months, says Heslin.

Make a plan. Once you decide to lose weight, wait at least two weeks before taking any action, advises Michael R. Lowe, Ph.D., associate professor of clinical psychology at Hahnemann University in Philadelphia. "Too many diets are impulsive," he says. "If you plan how you're going to diet, how you're going to work in your exercise, how you're going to eat out in different places, your commitment is likely to be stronger."

Keep a budget of daily fat, but don't forbid yourself to eat certain foods. A budget allows the flexibility to splurge on foods you crave as long as you keep the total fat count within limits. "There are no junk foods, provided you have balance and variety," says Dr. Drewnowski. "Go ahead and eat a burger. It won't kill you. Just don't have another one tomorrow."

Plot gradual changes. In the first weeks, eliminate eating in the car, for example, then banish eating in front of the TV. If you're drinking whole milk, ease into skim by first mixing whole with 2 percent. After a month, mix in 1 percent, and keep diluting until skim tastes good to you.

If you want to keep to an exercise schedule, Dr. Kushner recommends writing workouts into your calendar. "Appointments are powerful self-motivators for men," he says.

Weigh your progress. Weigh yourself every other day, advises Dr. Kushner. Men's weight doesn't fluctuate as wildly as women's, so you should see steady progress if you're sticking to your plan. Pat yourself on the back for any improvement, but don't judge yourself harshly if you suffer a setback. Even when you blow your diet a fifth of the time, that's an 80 percent success rate—good reason to keep going.

Follow these steps to banishing a potbelly, and you can retain the physique you had when you were 18 well into adulthood, according to Heslin. "There's no reason you shouldn't be able to wear the same jeans you had in your freshman year of college," she says.

—Richard Laliberte

Part 10

TAKING CARE
OF BUSINESS

The Essence of Control

*Ever wonder how you might get control over
your job, your stress, your time...your life?
Here are the answers.*

•••••••••••••••••••••

YOU SPEND MORE TIME at work than you do asleep in
your own bed. Where once you whispered sweet nothings in
your wife's ear, you now exchange urgent information: "Did
you pay the electric bill?" "Did the recyclable trash go out?"
"Did the plumber get the Little Mermaid doll out of the drain?"
Your daughter has taken to fantasizing that she is Shirley
Temple and you're her long-lost father, missing in action in the
Boer War.

This is not the life you set out to lead. It is, instead, a life careening wildly out of control, a life with a life of its own.

If this sounds familiar, it may not be your fault. Most of us are working more hours, and for all our toil in the corporate vineyard, our efforts don't always bear fruit. Our earnings are in a race with our expenses, and the expenses are winning. And because we have to work more just to keep even, free time is at a premium. Welcome to the 1990s.

"The average workweek has just exploded, to an average of over 46 hours," says time-management consultant and author Merrill Douglass. "I know managers and professionals who are working 50 and 60 hours. Top-level people often put in 60 to 70 hours, on average. We have millions of people out there whose lives consist of eating, sleeping, household maintenance and working, and I think they're hurting."

WELCOME TO CHAOS

Of course, you don't need a sour economy or a family to feel powerless in the face of daily responsibilities. Even in the best of times, your life may be chaotic. But the recent recession and the continuing financial difficulties underscore what is likely to be an important continuing theme in American life: the loss of control, and the need for more of it.

However, you *can* get your life back in order. Not just your work life, but your whole life. You can get control of your time so you have more of it to spend with family, with friends and by yourself. You can get control of the mounting stress so you have more peace of mind. And you can get control of your diet and exercise plans as well. Better still, you can achieve this kind of control by making a series of small changes.

The essence of control is a feeling, say the experts. You can't influence the outcome of every event in your life, explains clinical psychologist Ronald Nathan, Ph.D., coauthor of *The Doctors' Guide To Instant Stress Relief,* but you can *feel* in control. He describes this quality as an emotional hardiness, an almost chameleon-like adaptability.

This hardiness, he believes, is rooted in a sense of purpose. Purpose means having overriding goals, a comprehensive plan for your life that will see you through good times and bad. People who have this kind of long-range vision are able to see temporary setbacks for what they are; they know where they're going, and they aren't going to let anything stand in the way. "It all stems from a belief that you have real influence over what happens in your life through what you imagine, say or do," says Suzanne Ouellette Kobasa, Ph.D., a professor of psychology at the graduate school of the City University of New York.

A SENSE OF PURPOSE IS KEY

You can't instantaneously attain that belief. But even if it seems like your daily routine is an exercise in damage control, somewhere deep down you need a sense of purpose or the tools necessary to find it. Douglass, owner of Time Management Center in Marietta, Georgia, and coauthor of *Manage Your Time, Manage Your Work, Manage Yourself,* rec-

••

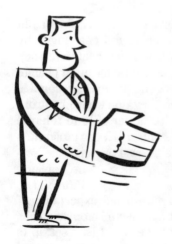

Lasting First Impressions

To make a solid impression among business associates, experts advise you to act confident—even if you don't feel that way. The reason: 80 percent of communication is attitude and body language; only 20 percent is verbal. Germaine Knapp, founder of a Rochester, New York, communications consulting firm, suggests the following tips for creating an aura of confidence.

■ Sit or stand erect.
■ Maintain eye contact.
■ Unfold your arms and legs.
■ To emphasize agreement, nod your head occasionally and say "yes."
■ To show command, sit at the head of a table, or stand while others are seated.

ommends following a clear and well-defined action plan that'll help you regain your sense of purpose and give you back your control.

To begin with, keep a journal in which you jot down what you do in every hour, in your work, family and personal life for a month. Once you've developed this sample one-month life map, look at the things you spend your time doing and separate them into things you love doing and things you don't. Then ask yourself: How much time do I spend doing the things I really want to do with my life? How can I rearrange my life to get more of what I want?

The experts stress that in identifying your desires, what you should be looking for are the kinds of things that would make you feel happy and fulfilled. This does not include short-term, transitory goals, like "Make megabucks" or "Become vice-president of the company," but rather things like "I want to work in a helping profession" or "I want to have more time in my life to be with my family."

"Once you've found that answer, the rest is relatively easy," says Douglass. "We spend so much time running around trying to figure out what to do. But we need to figure out what we want to *be* first."

Hardy people, those whom Dr. Nathan describes as in control of their lives, committed to goals and challenged by change, have one other telling characteristic: flexibility. They roll with the punches. They don't waste time trying to change what they can't change. "They have the ability to recognize when it's time to pull back or when they don't have control," says Dr. Ouellette Kobasa. "They're better able to tolerate ambiguity. People who don't feel in control just can't tolerate it when the world becomes unpredictable, as it often is."

FORGET FEAR OF FAILURE

"A lot of our stress has to do with failed expectations," adds Dr. Nathan, pointing out what may seem an obvious fact, but one we must all take to heart: "The world isn't set up to meet our expectations. We'd all be better off if we could remember that."

One of the major approaches to reducing stress, he adds, is to examine what your expectations are. If you expect to fix the garage-door opener, play golf, get a haircut and pick up your laundry all in one Saturday afternoon, you're going to feel out of control. Likewise, business and professional goals also need to be challenging but not out of reach. "And we have to change our expectations as the world changes," he says. "Often, our expectations lag behind where the world really is."

Sometimes circumstances really are overwhelming. There's too much to do, and not enough time to do it all. So you either adapt or find ways to reduce the pressures that are making you feel less than fully in control. Some general principles apply.

TAKE LITTLE BITES

First, don't bite off more than you can chew. Sounds simple, but it isn't always. Some men just can't say no. They have their fingers in every little pie, from negotiating multimillion-dollar contracts to choosing the color of the new office telephones. They do charity work. They're on the company softball team. They don't know how to stop.

Robert Dato, Ph.D., is a Wynnewood, Pennsylvania, psychoanalyst who helps executives learn to adapt to stress. He says he often sees men who are in way over their heads. "They come in and they tell me all the things they're doing. I try to understand all the pressures they don't need to be under," Dr. Dato says. He helps them decide what's best for them, which usually means reducing pressure and increasing adaptability in stressful situations. "When they do this, they get great relief, but it's like they need the permission of a therapist, a father figure," says Dr. Dato. "I tell them it's okay."

Of course, you don't need a therapist to tell you when you're doing too much. You probably already know. Nor should you need anyone's permission to pull back but your own. If you can't go cold turkey, try dropping one activity at a time until the pressure's off.

It may be easy to drop all your extracurricular activities, but it's not so simple to tell your boss you just don't feel like doing accounts payable today. Still, even at work, there are ways to extricate yourself tactfully when you're overloaded. If you do it with enough skill, says Dr. Nathan, your boss will think you're saying no for his own good: "Say, 'I'm overcom-

• •

NEAT LITTLE TIMESAVERS

Here are some nifty tricks to help you gain better control of your life.

■ Hang a key rack near the front door and make it a habit to put your keys there as soon as you walk in. You'll never again have to frantically search for them when you're already running late.

■ Get up 15 minutes earlier in the morning. Then, if anything goes wrong, you won't have to deal with being late on top of it. Likewise, plan to leave 15 minutes earlier than you usually do for appointments so you won't have to rush.

■ Lay out your clothes, fill the coffee machine and check your briefcase before you go to bed. Mornings are so much easier when all the details are arranged.

■ Pay all your bills on the same day each month. Ideally this should be the same day you get your bank statement, so you can reconcile it at the same time. File all bills that arrive after this date in a central location to be paid next month.

■ Use pickup and delivery services whenever possible. You'll save time, and in many cases you'll save money as well when you take into account the cost of driving to get the paper or the dry cleaning.

• •

mitted, and I can't really do that justice,' " Dr. Nathan recommends. "Say, 'I'm flattered that you asked, but I wouldn't want to agree to do something for you if I really didn't have the time to do a good job.' "

Another approach, for bosses with harder heads, is to offer options, says Douglass. "Tell him, 'I'd really like to do this for you, but I can't do it without giving up something else. Which of these things would you most like me to do?' Most bosses will take the hint."

GET FIT

Along with emotional hardiness, physical fitness can go a long way toward improving your sense of well-being. Clearly, exercise benefits the body and makes you hardier, says Dr.

• •

■ Set priorities. Write your day's tasks, in order of importance, on a series of sticky notes. When you complete a task, peel off the note and crumple it up with a feeling of accomplishment.

■ Avoid business lunches when possible. Use the time as a psychological break, a time to balance out the morning and afternoon.

■ Use a tape recorder for your correspondence. It's twice as efficient as dictation or longhand.

■ To make Mondays easier, take the last hour of every Friday to straighten up your office. Write reminders to yourself for Monday morning. Also, save a couple of your more pleasurable tasks for Monday.

■ The average executive wastes 288 hours a year in unnecessary meetings. Go into meetings with a clear objective. Beforehand, ask yourself questions like "Do I need to reach a decision about something?" "Do I want to share information?" Ask yourself if you could handle things more easily in a memo or by phone.

■ Plan a way to avoid interruptions. Set aside a time each day when you can work without distraction. Make sure everyone on your staff knows when that time is. Then close the door.

• •

Ouellette Kobasa, but, she adds, "it has something to do, too, with what's going on in your head. People who can get up from their desks and take a ten-minute walk feel better about themselves than those people who say, 'I can't ever leave my desk.' That ten minutes of walking is just for you. It is also a time for some reflection. While you're out walking, you can see a problem for what it is, and you often come back with a much better perspective."

Exercise done outside of work is also very helpful, she says, because it puts you into contact with other people. Social support is another key element in the development of that elusive thing called hardiness. "The human organism is a complex thing," says Ouellette Kobasa, "and we're more resistant to stress when we have this combination of social, psychological and biological factors working in our favor."

One unscheduled activity that intrudes on your sense of well-being throughout the day is worry. And the more you worry, the more you feel that you're not in control. Worry overwhelms all reason. And even as you budget time for work and play, worry has free rein. One solution Dr. Nathan recommends is to set aside a formal time each day for worry.

"Sometimes we worry superstitiously, as if worrying will control the future," Dr. Nathan says. "People are under the illusion that they're somehow planning what to do. But are they planning or worrying?"

If you're really planning, he suggests that you pull out the pad and pencil and write down what you're going to do. But if you're really just worrying, nothing's being accomplished. You're giving yourself a false sense of control.

SCHEDULE YOUR WORRYING

Research suggests that setting aside time for worry—a half hour toward the end of each day—actually decreases the amount of worry by an average of 35 percent, thus increasing your sense of well-being.

Finally, whenever you're able, try to accentuate the positive. So maybe your Alfa-Romeo needs a $1,100 transmission job. Maybe the kids need braces and your cat is allergic to fleas. Okay, so the IRS has sent you a notice that you're being audited. All true, and all pretty gruesome. On the other hand, you're healthy. Your marriage is good. Your kids think you're God and you could *afford* the fancy car in the first place. "The key," says Dr. Nathan, "is to identify areas of your life where you *do* have control."

In the meantime, hang in there. As someone once said, you can't smooth out the surf, but you can learn to ride the waves.

—Jeff Meade

Execu-Pains

As if you didn't know, the repressed urge to punch or kick somebody results in muscular stresses. If that somebody happens to be at your place of work, here's what to do.

•••••••••••••••••••••••

DAVE HOWARD IS ONE of the most stressed-out people I know, and I know a *lot* of stressed-out people. In the past five years, Dave has had three middle-management jobs shot out from under him for reasons beyond his control. And each job seems more stressful than the last. Most recently, he was with the U.S. branch of a Japanese firm. To meet incredibly tight and unforgiving production deadlines, it was essential that he communicate closely with a man who didn't speak very good English. After months of trying to boost the guy's language skills by chatting about women and whatnot, there came a crisis. "I told him the schedule wasn't working, we had to ship in three days, and he was getting way behind," Dave recalls. "I said, 'Do you understand?' And he said, 'Girlfriend?' "

Griping about this stuff over a not-so-happy-hour beer helps Dave get through. But it does nothing for the aches he gets all over—in his jaw, neck and shoulders (which often lead to headaches) and in his lower back and legs. Sometimes the pains hit him singly; sometimes they gang up on him. He's a walking—rather, *sitting*—textbook on what Richard M. Bachrach, D.O., calls execu-pains.

As medical director of the Center for Sports and Osteopathic Medicine in New York, Dr. Bachrach sees the same gallery of minor aches and pains all the time among his white-collar clientele. Often the underlying problem is a lack of exercise or bottled-up aggression, he says. "Guys who don't get enough physical activity can't diffuse the energy that builds up from day-to-day frustrations. The repressed urge to punch or kick somebody results directly in muscular stresses, particularly among lower-level executives who have a lot of responsibility but no control over their jobs."

CLENCH YOUR FIST

To get an idea of where neck pain actually comes from, clench your fist and visualize what's going on inside. Muscles are hard, contracted, pressing against the skin. These muscles also push against nerves, and over time those nerves can become irritated, explains Richard M. Linchitz, M.D., medical director of the Pain Alleviation Center in Roslyn, New York. Different people express their tension in different parts of the body. "Some get ulcers, some develop high blood pressure, some will get a heart attack in 20 years—and some get neck pains and tension headaches," says Dr. Linchitz. "In certain people there seems to be a kind of constitutional predisposition—a weakness—to muscular pain."

Often, the weakness stems from an injury (which itself could be stress-related—tense muscles are less supple). My friend Dave's problems began when a nerve became pinched by a swollen disk while running. It healed, but slowly. He stopped exercising, which set off a spiraling degeneration: Lack of activity made him more susceptible to stress, which made his back feel worse, which kept him awake nights, which left him exhausted—making his back feel worse. Then the aches and pains began to spread. In severe cases, this kind of progression can lead to a chronic condition called fibromyalgia that lasts for months or years and virtually incapacitates people.

But it needn't be so. "These pains are very interrelated, and we can manage them ourselves, without expensive or time-consuming treatments," says Dr. Bachrach. The best remedy is to relieve the stress itself, either by avoiding anxiety-provoking situations or by tapping a variety of relaxation techniques. But there are also physical ways to soothe pains where they live—in the muscles.

Prescription number one is exercise. "In some cases, working the muscle that's in pain ultimately can be the best thing for it, despite the usual wisdom of not doing something that hurts," Dr. Linchitz says. (But don't push pained muscles too far. It's important that exercises be moderate and properly performed.) Stretching to relieve stiffness can help keep pains from ever hitting, but if you hurt in a particular area, you should perform a therapeutic stretch at least three times a day. Here's a guide to the six most common execu-pains and the simplest, most effective tips for easing them.

HEAD AND NECK ACHES

They almost always go together. Common causes are cradling a phone with your shoulder or craning your neck to view a computer screen. That pain in the neck often radiates upward, creating a band of tightness from the base of the skull or around the forehead.

1. Sitting erect in a chair, let your chin fall gently to your chest, allowing the weight of your head to stretch muscles at the back of the neck. Keep the neck relaxed, and hold for 30 seconds. Next, lean your head back gently and look at the ceiling for 30 seconds. (Caution: Older men, 65 years and up, may feel faint or pass out when they do this stretch. Check with your doctor first.)

2. With your left hand, grip the bottom of the chair you're sitting on so that your left shoulder pulls down slightly, then lean your head gently to the right. Hold for 30 seconds. Repeat, opposite side.

JAW SORENESS

This problem is typically characterized by pain on one side of the face shooting into the head. People under pressure have a tendency to clench and grind their teeth, which can lead to a jaw malady called temporomandibular joint (TMJ) disorder. "But a lot of so-called TMJ problems are really due to muscular tension on one side of the jaw," says Dr. Linchitz. "That creates an imbalance, and the muscle acts as if there's a problem in the joint itself."

1. Open your mouth about halfway and gently swivel the lower jaw right and left, moving it continuously for about 30 seconds.

2. Bring your lower jaw forward and up in front of the upper jaw ten times before a meal and another ten times before bed.

3. To keep from clenching your teeth, hold your jaw open slightly so upper and lower teeth are separated. Rest your tongue lightly against the roof of your mouth without pressing it against the front teeth. With practice, this may become habitual, reducing the urge to clench or grind.

SHOULDER PAIN

Most shoulder soreness comes from irregular use of or physical abuse to muscles and tendons, but with stress, neck pains can irritate the nerves that lead to the arms, allowing pain to radiate to the shoulders.

1. Bring your left arm in front of your body, across your chest. Hook your right arm under your left elbow and pull your left arm across your chest. Hold for 30 seconds and release. Repeat, opposite side.

2. Raise your left arm straight up and grab the top or side of a door frame. Holding the frame, walk through the door until you feel muscles stretch gently. Hold for 30 seconds and release. Repeat with your right arm.

3. Reach up to your side at a 45-degree angle, taking hold of a door frame with your left hand. Gently twist your body to the right, away from the raised arm. Hold for 30 seconds and release. Repeat with your right arm.

4. Hold one arm straight out to the side, elbow bent at 90 degrees, as if taking an oath. Grab the side of a door frame with your raised hand and walk through the door until muscles stretch gently. Hold for 30 seconds. Release, then repeat with the other arm.

BACKACHES

The back is particularly vulnerable because muscles here do most of the work of supporting the body when you're sitting. "If you don't have a good chair, you're dead," says Dave, my stressed-out friend. But even if your company springs for the latest ergonomic wonder, you should change position a lot, stand when you're on the phone and stretch frequently. When pain hits, if it's mild, try these stretches. (For severe back pain, consult your doctor.)

1. Grab the doorknobs on both sides of an open door. Keeping your arms straight in front of you and your feet flat on the floor, squat as low as you can while pulling on the knobs. Hold for 30 seconds, then stand up. Caution: Don't do this exercise if you have bad knees.

2. While sitting in your chair, grab one knee with both hands and bring it to your chest. Hold for 15 to 30 seconds. Repeat with the other knee.

LEG PAIN

Pain often starts in the lower back and shoots downward. Leg pains are often called sciatica, a condition that may signal serious problems from a herniated disk. However, more than 90 percent of sciatica-like pain isn't true sciatica, but minor pain (usually in the buttocks and upper leg) caused by prolonged sitting. (Don't get alarmed unless the pain extends below the knee or persists for several days.)

To stretch buttocks muscles, sit erect in a chair and cross your left leg over your right, ankle on knee. Cup your left knee with your left hand and your left ankle with your right hand. Simultaneously pull your knee and ankle toward your right shoulder until you feel muscles stretch slightly. Hold for 30 seconds and release. Repeat with your right leg.

Stretches like these helped get Dave back on track. For his particular problem, his doctor also recommended taking up swimming, an activity which doesn't strain his still-sensitive back. He'll always be nervous about job security, but he's now

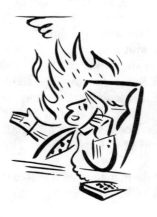

If You Can't Stand the Heat...You Know the Rest

In rising to the top, the ability to handle stress is more important than a born talent for management, says *Fit for Success* author James Rippe, M.D. A chief prescription for coping with stress: exercise. When the heat is on, conditioned bodies pump out less nerve-racking adrenaline and more endorphins, the brain chemicals that promote feelings of well-being.

comfortably ensconsed in a stable wing of a stable company. He says his pains are becoming less frequent and less intense. The stress is still there, but he had to hang up before he could finish telling me about it: His boss was coming and he didn't want to have to explain exactly what he was doing talking to a reporter on company time.

—*Richard Laliberte*

John Henry Had It Wrong

If you believe that simply putting your nose to the grindstone will allow you to succeed, take a lesson from the man who died trying.

• •

By NOW, MOST OF US have found out that there's no such thing as an A for effort. In the real world of real work, effort doesn't count a whole lot in the absence of results. Still, the notion that we'll always be rewarded for working hard is one that some men carry with them all their lives. It's all mixed up with popular American myths about rising from rags to riches, from some humble shanty to the White House. "I can do anything," we're encouraged to believe. "The sky's the limit."

Social scientists have come up with a name for this kind of hard-work-beats-all reasoning: *John Henryism.*

You remember the story: John Henry was the best steel-driving man on the railroad. When a machine came along to do his job, he swore he could outperform steam power any day. In a contest, John Henry indeed beat the machine, but then collapsed with a ruptured blood vessel in his head. Not exactly a clear victory.

Today, John Henry is the middle manager who sets out irrationally to leapfrog a grade level in the company by adding projects to a plate that's already too full. He's the entrepreneur who resolves this year to crack a business market that's long resisted his best efforts. He's the man who sets out to buy a house he can barely afford, despite a downturn in his business.

"John Henry epitomizes a spirit of hard work and determination against all odds," says E. C. McKetney, Ph.D., an epidemiologist at the University of California, Berkeley. "And John Henryism is a belief that simply putting your nose to the grindstone and doing things on your own will allow you to succeed no matter what."

NEVER SAYING NO

It's not just working hard that makes for a John Henry. It can also be striving unrealistically for goals that you lack the money, the time, the talent or even the social connections to accomplish.

Over time, this approach to the world can kill you just as it did the man the syndrome was named after. The stress of working long hours and never saying no in situations where you can't make a difference may eventually wreck your mental or physical health, says Salvatore Maddi, Ph.D., professor of psychology at the University of California, Irvine, and president of the Hardiness Institute, a stress-management firm.

Studies find that stress plays a role in the onset of 90 percent of mental disorders, and some medical professionals estimate that 60 percent of all visits to a doctor are stress-related. "You use up your body's resources, and your immune system turns to mush," Dr. Maddi asys. Wearing down the body can eventually hasten the progress of life-threatening problems such as heart disease and cancer. Studies among low-income, uneducated, rural blacks—people whose resources for accomplishing their goals are especially low—find that men who believe most strongly that hard work and determination will overcome obstacles have higher rates of hypertension than men who are more laid back.

How can you tell if you're a John Henry? According to Sherman James, Ph.D., the University of Michigan epidemiologist who created the John Henryism concept, you'll have a bedrock of certain core attitudes. When the going gets tough, a

John Henry wants to work harder and will stick with a job until it's completely done, always managing to find a way to do the things he really needs to get done. In the face of setbacks, he *never* loses sight of his goals. He's fiercely individualistic and likes doing things that other people thought couldn't be done—and doing them his way. He may also be a little bit overbearing, sometimes feeling that he's the only one who can do a job right.

OVERCOMING INSECURITY

Ironically, these very qualities, in moderation, are what lead to career success. "Managers love people like that," observes Howard Mase, Ph.D., a vice-president at Metropolitan Life Personal Insurance. "They stay all hours, work on weekends, do things nobody else will and don't like to take vacations." Like John Henry himself, they're willing to keep pounding away at problems, even if it kills them.

There's nothing inherently troublesome about having a hard-work ethic, Dr. James says. Problems start when it's combined with unreasonable ambition.

• •

You Can't Hide Those Lying Eyes

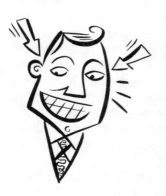

Ever wonder whether one of your associates was smiling at you out of friendship or to hide the fact that he hates your guts? Now you don't have to be a mind reader to tell. The trick is to check the skin folds around the eyes, says psychologist Paul Ekman of the University of California, San Francisco. True smiles of enjoyment are recognized by a characteristic wrinkling of the skin around the eyes. Lying smiles can be detected by a tightening of the muscles around the mouth and narrowing of the lips.

"If these men accomplish one set of goals, they set higher ones," says Stephen Weinstein, Ph.D., clinical professor of psychiatry and human behavior at Thomas Jefferson University Medical College in Philadelphia. "It's an endless cycle, and they never feel they accomplish much of anything. The result is stress, disappointment and frustration."

Psychologists say men often work hard just for the sake of work because they don't feel good about themselves if they're not productive. Deep down, it may have to do with feelings they got from their parents that their worth in the world is measured by what they do, not by who they are. Working hard, according to this view, becomes a way for them to control affection and gain the admiration of other people.

In this respect, John Henry types bear a resemblance to people with Type-A personalities, whose hard-driving, aggressive and often hostile behavior make them particularly stress-prone. John Henrys lack many of the hallmark Type-A characteristics—they're not likely to express anger forcefully, for example—but both personalities have an overwhelming need for absolute control over their lives, says Dr. Maddi. "For them to assess a situation and say, 'I can't do anything' is the worst thing in the world for them," he says. "They'll never reach that conclusion. They'll just try harder. The trouble is, they won't always be successful."

FINDING PEACE

Consider the case of Lee Atwater, the late chairman of the Republican Party. When he learned he had inoperable cancer, the 39-year-old Atwater marshalled his staff and instructed them to explore every possibility for finding a cure. He was determined that the disease would not beat him. Whether his frustration hastened his death is anybody's guess, but eventually he came to terms with the fact that the matter was out of his hands. That, according to his own account, is when he began to find some peace.

So it is with the rest of us, psychologists say. What we need—and what John Henrys lack—is to accept that yes, we can accomplish a lot by dint of our own effort, but some obstacles in life are as immovable as the Rockies. So instead of butting your head against the stone, go around it. Instead of working so hard to overcome your weaknesses, start doing more things that accentuate your strengths.

How do you know when a goal is unrealistic? It sounds trite, but you won't know until you try. "Goals should always be challenging," says Cliff Mangan, Ph.D., a psychologist at Temple University Counseling Center in Philadelphia. "But you have to ask yourself if what you're doing is getting you toward that goal."

If your goal is to rise two grade levels in your company, break your approach into smaller, more manageable goals— rising first to the next-highest level, for example, or cultivating the social contacts that may boost your ascent. Give yourself a specific, reasonable amount of time for these developments to occur.

If your efforts don't seem to pay off, try another approach, such as getting more training or education, suggests Dr. Maddi. "Persistence can be helpful, but you need to see clearly what can be changed and what can't," he says. When you run out of ideas, it's time to get out of the steam engine's way and find something else to challenge.

—*Richard Laliberte*

Surviving Success

A counselor to the rich and powerful tells how to keep from hitting bottom when you reach the top.

••••••••••••••••••••••

YOU EXPECT TO MAKE a few sacrifices on your way to the top. The hope is that you'll be more than compensated for the price of success when you reach that big payoff at the peak.

However, many men discover that the cost is just too steep. They've reaped material rewards but feel they've been emotionally swindled in the process. "Success is one of the most psychologically disruptive experiences a person can endure," says Steven Berglas, Ph.D., a clinical psychologist and management consultant at Harvard Medical School, and author of *The Success Syndrome: Hitting Bottom When You Reach the Top.*

It's largely a matter of feeling isolated from other people, says Dr. Berglas, and the more successful you are, the less likely it is that others will take your emotional needs seriously.

Is it possible to reach your career goals with your emotional health intact? Dr. Berglas says yes. In his practice at the Executive Stress Clinic in Chestnut Hill, Massachusetts, he counsels achievers on their problems and how to overcome them. We asked him to share some of his insights.

Q. It seems as though people don't have a good understanding of what success is really like. What are some myths about success?

A. The major myth is that career success will transform your personal life. People honestly believe that if they are good at their job they will have friends and lovers as a result. There is no correlation. In fact, there's an antagonism between achieving career success and achieving emotional satisfaction. The skills and attributes necessary for one contradict the other.

Q. Why is that?

A. The traditional route to the top is through the acquisition of wealth and power, not affection. When clients start therapy, I try to get them to discover how they came to depend on financial rewards to secure all forms of gratification. Then we explore what I call the Law of Inverse Business Effects: how actions that advance careers—using the backs of others as stepping stones, for example, or choosing friends on the basis of what they'll do for your career—typically derail relationships.

Highly successful people are often prone to severe bouts of depression. They have an overwhelming sense of emptiness and isolation. If you feel all you've got going for you is money, then everyone around you, including your spouse, seems to be after you for what you can give them rather than who you are. Having no real interpersonal relationships has incredibly devastating effects psychologically.

Q. What are some other problems that go along with success?

A. There's a "halo effect," where the person who's successful in one realm is presumed competent and talented in all others. That generates inordinate expectations, and people really aren't equipped to live up to them. Buzz Aldrin is one of my favorite examples. He had a nervous breakdown after walking on the moon. He was a great astronaut and a great military man, but a horrible hero. He was uncomfortable around people. He was overwhelmed by the social adoration, the expectation that he could also be an after-dinner speaker or chairman of the board.

Another belief about success is that if you do "X" today, you should be able to do "X plus one" tomorrow. It's a constant upward spiral of expectations that no human can live up to. But for men who are dependent on success for their identity, there's no quitting. Ultimately, they'll sacrifice relationships to focus more energy on their careers.

Q. How do people come to recognize these problems in themselves?

A. Let's speak in terms of physical warning signs. The first thing people do is self-medicate—they'll drink more coffee and alcohol, take sleeping aids and often try harder drugs, trying to provide themselves with an "up." The second symptom is an irritability with the family. The third is adultery, as individuals blame partners for their failure to feel upbeat about life. The fourth symptom is trying to seek adventure— buying jet skis or doing an adventurous trip like Outward Bound, for example. When those magic bullets don't work, often they come to psychotherapy and realize there's been a dearth of appropriate rewards.

Q. You've written that this often takes place between the age of 38 and 42. What's so special about that time in a man's life?

A. When I say that, I'm talking about fast trackers. People in the middle lane would experience this around 50. It's whenever material reinforcers lose their value. You find it does no good to buy a new Rolex or a new Mercedes or a new boat.

You just run out of toys. And at the same time you're losing your taste for material things, you discover your inability to achieve emotional and personal satisfaction. It's when you realize you've gotten there and it ain't what it's cracked up to be.

Promotions are often a trigger. People assume a promotion will change everything—that now they'll have time for their wife, they'll be a better father, they'll go back to playing basketball at the YMCA, and they'll finally feel great.

Nothing of the sort happens. Their interpersonal relationships don't improve, and their anxieties get worse because they have to live up to more expectations. The money and perks make no difference. They move into the corner office, wake up two weeks later and find nothing has improved.

Q. So are you saying there are no benefits to being a success?

A. Not at all. Successful men have opportunities that others do not. If you can clear up your debts, feel secure that your job won't be taken away and aren't concerned with basic self-preservation in your career, you can begin to look at who you are and where you fit into the world. This kind of security allows you to explore relationships, develop your spirituality, and figure out where you stand in the world and what it's all about. It's wonderful to be successful if you take advantage of the opportunities you've created.

Q. What does it take to reach the top and stay psychologically healthy?

A. In the studies I've done, the people who are healthy when they reach the top have a strong cultural or religious involvement. I didn't expect to find this church component, but it really is there. They don't necessarily believe strongly in God or the tenets of a church. They don't say the rosary or don't keep a kosher home, but they believe in Catholicism, believe in Judaism, believe in their ethnic heritage.

They also have an intact family, and they engage in some form of mentoring. There's a sense of wanting to bring others along, a sense of nurturing, of being a giver. They engage in volunteerism that takes hands-on "sweat equity" in a project, not just saying, "Here's $100,000, put my name on a building." They're very involved, but they don't need monuments.

Q. Can you cite some examples of men who have actually done this?

A. The best one is Peter Lynch of the Magellan Fund. Richest guy on Wall Street and he walks away to spend time with his wife and daughters. He's also involved with the church and the alumni association at Boston College. Another example is Thomas Monaghan of Domino's Pizza. He's one of the richest men in America, and he's cutting back in his midforties to do missionary work for the church.

Q. What else can we do on the way up?

A. The major thing I advocate is systematically trading off material gratifications for interpersonal rewards. If a move will take you away from a place where you're starting to root and to develop a social network, pass up the 10 percent raise and realize you're being paid back in other ways. If a promotion involves travel and you don't want to travel, pass up the promotion. Another one will come along.

I also advocate entering organizations outside your work where you can be an "Indian," not a "chief." It's no good being an executive in a community softball league if you're also an executive at work—it isn't going to permit you to develop the interpersonal contacts that make you feel good about who you are. But when you're a drone, people come to know you as a person. Peer groups like the Young Presidents Organization can have the same effect because members can relate to one another as people—everybody's as rich as everybody else, so they're not there for the hustle.

Q. What about family life? Do the same principles apply?

A. Exactly. I see plenty of high-powered types who don't know how to stop behaving like executives. They come home, sit at the dining room table and hold a board meeting, with progress reports from each child as though he were a little subsidiary. This is probably the biggest problem they confront. They have to learn to be a peer in the family, not always a superstar, to abandon competency as a method of gaining intimacy.

The easiest way to do it is through what's called a strategic pratfall effect. You need to show vulnerability to your kids and your spouse. Tell a child, "I'm afraid of those computers you're learning with" or "I don't know that foreign language you're studying." When your son comes to you to talk about his fears, don't say, "You need to be strong like me." That's another distancing technique. It intimidates him and tells him that it's not okay to be human. Instead say, "When I was your age, this was something I went through."

You have to differentiate *liking,* which you want from your family, from *respect,* which you want from your colleagues. You don't tell your colleagues you're scared. You definitely tell your kids.

Q. What's the moral of the story?

A. Love and work are the key to mental health, and in America, we've really denigrated the role of love. By love I mean love of God, love of community, love of principles, love of people. Romantic love, too.

I advise tons of companies to let their young executives teach, mentor, get involved with community outreach. The corporation will be polishing its image better than any media consultant would, and the executives will feel more like people. This would be a tremendous benefit.

—Richard Laliberte

Part 11

ASK
MEN'S HEALTH

The 20 Most Pressing
Questions on Men's Minds

From New England to Florida to California,
here's what guys have been wondering about.

••••••••••••••••••••••

The following letters are among the many hundreds I get
every year as editor of *Men's Health* magazine. Why these 20?
I felt these were awfully representative of the kinds of things
on most guys' minds. Maybe on yours?

—*Mike Lafavore*

SMOKING ON THE RUN

Q. They say balance is one of the keys to healthy living. One way I keep my life in balance is by allowing myself some self-indulgent activities on the weekend. One of these is a couple of cigarettes. I console myself with the promise of making up for it on my weekday-morning runs. Does the increase in lung capacity I get from running help reverse the negative effects of the smoking?

—Y.H., Burlington, Vt.

A. Close, but no cigar. Although aerobic exercise can make your oxygen processing more efficient, it does little to offset the effects of smoking. Tobacco smoke, which contains more than 4,000 chemicals (43 of them known carcinogens), hinders the lungs' ability to filter out obstructions that can irritate and scar their lining. Unfortunately, exercise does little to eliminate the carcinogens or reduce the irritation caused by smoking.

About the only good news we have for you is that the hazards of smoking are usually dose-responsive: the more you smoke, the greater your risk of falling prey to smoking-related ills like lung cancer. Since you seem to be keeping your smoking to a minimum, your risk of lung disease may not be so great. But why play high-stakes poker with your health?

VASECTOMY REVERSAL

Q. I had a vasectomy at age 31, and last year at age 34, I had it reversed. Now I have a low sperm count and my sperm has low motility, but my urologist says I still have a chance of becoming fertile again. Is there anything I can do to improve my odds?

—M.G., New York, N.Y.

A. It depends on how low your sperm count and motility are, but the prognosis is good for men who have had a vasectomy reversed within five years, says reversal specialist Marc Goldstein, M.D., director of the Male Reproduction and Microsurgery Unit at New York Hospital–Cornell Medical Center. "In the 400 reversals I've done, 98 percent of the men who had their reversal within five years of their vasectomy regained their fertility and 75 percent managed to get their partners pregnant within two years."

Although the numbers drop a bit in men who wait up to ten years, they are still very good—95 percent and 62 percent, respectively.

Even though you still have a low sperm count and low motility, you may be fertile. Have your urologist test you to see if you have developed antisperm antibodies. Men still produce sperm after a vasectomy, but the body has to break them down internally, so it develops antibodies that attack and destroy the sperm as if it were a foreign substance. If antibodies are present, ask your urologist about treatment with prednisone or a similar steroid that suppresses the antibody response. Another option is to have your sperm "washed" with special chemicals to remove the antibodies. The "cleaned" sperm would then be injected directly into your partner's uterus when she is fertile. In vitro fertilization may also succeed, even for men with exceedingly low counts, as long as their sperm are healthy and mobile.

If none of these alternatives works, you may want to ask your urologist about having another reversal to remove any possible narrowing or leaks in your vas deferens.

VITAMIN CONFUSION

Q. Is it a good idea to take multivitamins, or is it better to take individual supplements? My multivitamin provides 100 percent of the RDA for most vitamins and minerals, but I'm worried that taking large amounts of many nutrients every day might hurt my system. What do you think?

—P.J., Cupertino, Calif.

A. Although any dietitian will tell you it is best to meet all your nutritional needs by eating a balanced diet, a standard multivitamin can be a safe and adequate supplement for athletes or people on the go. "Multivitamins are fine for you if you're not eating a wide variety of foods and feel you may be missing certain nutrients," says Martin Yadrick, a registered dietitian at the University of Kansas Medical Center.

He cautions against daily use of a multivitamin that supplies more than 100 percent of the Recommended Dietary Allowance (RDA) for many nutrients, "especially when you're talking about fat-soluble vitamins like A, D and E, which are stored in the liver and aren't easily excreted by the body."

As for individual supplements, most dietitians advise against these, since they usually supply megadoses of vitamins or minerals, which are far in excess of the RDA.

For a more specific or intense supplementation plan, check with your doctor or a registered dietitian.

SPICY DIET

Q. Does eating spicy foods like jalapeño peppers pose any health problems?

—A.R., North Hollywood, Calif.

A. Not at all. Studies have shown that spicy foods are harmless, despite the very real feeling that they are burning the lips, mouth, throat and stomach, according to Samuel Klein, M.D., associate professor of medicine in the division of gastroenterology at the University of Texas Medical Branch. The burning sensation is caused by a chemical in the peppers (capsaicin), which tricks the nerves into signaling the brain that they are being burnt.

Spicy foods can and do cause some men heartburn. Liquid antacids made from aluminum magnesium hydroxide will put out the fire.

LOST IN A FOG

Q. Although my health club has a sauna and a steam room, nobody there can tell me the particular benefits of each one. Can you defog this mystery for me?

—J.R., New York, N.Y.

A. "There are really no therapeutic advantages or disadvantages to either one," says W. Larry Kenney, Ph.D., associate professor of applied physiology at Pennsylvania State University. Saunas rely on dry heat (up to 280° F). Steam rooms fill with, well, steam and reach temperatures of 220°.

Advocates claim that both can help stimulate weight loss, cleanse toxins from the body, clear up skin conditions and decrease recovery time after exercise.

As appealing as these claims sound, there's little physiological evidence to support them. Still, Dr. Kenney and others agree that sitting in a sauna or a steam room does *feel* good and will relax you. Doing so may be beneficial, from a psychological point of view, after a grueling workout.

Which is better, steam or sauna? "They both work equally well; it's just a matter of personal preference," says Dr. Kenney.

One word of caution: After a strenuous workout, your body temperature is already elevated, so be sure to drink plenty of fluids and cool off for 15 to 20 minutes before a sauna or steam.

HOT HAIR

Q. I'm 30 years old, and every morning I blow-dry my hair before going to work. Now my hair is beginning to thin out on the top, and my wife says that I should stop blow-drying it, since this damages my hair and causes it to fall out faster. Is this true or just a lot of hot air?

—*S.A., Taos, N.M.*

A. Although blow-drying can make hair overdry and more susceptible to splitting, it will not itself cause hair to fall out. Combing or brushing too hard, however, can lead to hair loss, and men frequently do brush their hair vigorously while blow-drying, says *Men's Health* advisor John Romano, M.D., dermatologist at New York Hospital–Cornell Medical Center. He says if you blow-dry carefully and brush gently, you'll have no hair loss. First, towel dry your hair to remove excess water. Then blow-dry, keeping the unit six to ten inches away from your hair and running it at a low to medium setting. While drying, use fingers, not a comb, to get your hair going where you want. Then *gently* style with a wide-tooth comb or brush.

BOXERS OR BRIEFS?

Q. I've heard that wearing regular briefs can make a guy sterile. If this is true, would it be better to switch to boxer shorts?

—*M.D., Sacramento, Calif.*

A. Wearing briefs, even if they're tight fitting, will not produce any fertility problems. Just ask Jim Palmer or his two kids. Over the years, researchers have theorized that briefs may interfere with a man's sperm production by holding the testicles too close to the body and thus elevating their temperature, but no studies have definitively shown this to be the case, says Jack Jaffe, M.D., medical director of the Potency Recovery Center in Van Nuys, California. "The majority of men today wear briefs and don't have any fertility problems. But if one of my patients comes to me with fertility problems and wants to try making the switch, I tell him to go ahead. It's like eating chicken soup if you have a cold—can't hurt."

FUZZY KISSES

Q. For years my wife has been nagging me to shave off my mustache because, she says, it feels like a broom when I kiss her. But I like it. Is there anything I can do to soften it so I stop rubbing her the wrong way?

—*S.P., San Jose, Calif.*

A. Get a trim. "Most mustaches get in the way because they're too long," says Peter Bradley, general manager of Vidal Sassoon Salons in the United States. "It doesn't have to be big and bushy to be a problem; even a little extra can make your wife feel as if she just kissed your power sander instead of you." Also, avoid washing your mustache with regular soap. It will leave a residue that can make your mustache especially coarse. Instead, treat it like the hair on your head: Shampoo it, then rinse and apply a moisturizing conditioner. Allow the conditioner to stay on for 60 to 90 seconds and rinse again. If this doesn't make you a softie, check your local hair salon before getting out the razor; some carry special moisturizers for facial hair.

HONESTY AT WORK

Q. Recently I was asked to gather information about a counterpart who works for one of my company's chief competitors. The method I was asked to use was at best unethical and in all likelihood illegal. When I informed my boss about my concerns, he implied that failure to do "my job" could result in being fired. What's the best way to handle the situation?

—*T.M., Cleveland, Ohio*

A. We agree with Jiminy Cricket on this one: You have to let your conscience be your guide. But listening to a lawyer wouldn't hurt, either. "What some people consider to be illegal or unethical may actually be within the boundaries of the law, so it might be wise for you to discuss your situation with someone who knows," suggests Bob Brady, publisher of *Business and Legal Reports* and an attorney who specializes in employment law. "Maybe there's a way you can do what was asked of you without having to violate your conscience.

"If you refuse to compromise your principles and are fired as a result, you could sue your employer and possibly win," adds Brady. "But you would have to prove that you were terminated because of it—and that would be difficult." It's unlikely that the reason given for your termination would be that you were "too honest."

Besides the difficulty in proving your case, suing isn't a smart career move. Even if you won, once word got out that you sued your employer—and word would get out—it would be very difficult to get another job. No matter how noble your reasons, jobs don't come easy to those with a history of taking their employers to court.

In the meantime, we advise you start looking for another job—ASAP. Any boss who would fire you for your scruples would fire you for any number of lame reasons. "If you're an ethical person working for an unethical boss, the best long-term advice is to find another boss," says Brady.

TROUBLED BACK

Q. Having had a bad back for many years, I've always been told that swimming is the best exercise for me. However, I'm not too fond of swimming and was wondering if there are any back-friendly exercises for us landlubbers.

—*P.B., Endicott, N.Y.*

A. Trainers recommend swimming to anyone with a bad back because the exercise provides the double benefit of strength and aerobic conditioning without much joint and bone pounding. But swimming isn't right for everyone. "No one activity works equally well for all those with bad backs, so we usually have to experiment," says Tom Lorren, a physical therapist and director of rehabilitation at the Texas Back Institute in Dallas. He's found that choosing the right exercise depends on knowing the *kind* of back injury you have. If you have a disk problem, you might try walking, or cross-country skiing on an indoor simulator. If you have spinal stenosis (narrowing of the column that surrounds the spinal cord), your best bet is cycling or rowing. If your problem is a garden-variety muscle strain or spasm, walking or cross-country ski machines usually work best.

Before embarking on any exercise plan, have your back problem diagnosed by an orthopedist or physical therapist. Then ask him what exercise choices would be best for you.

REDNECK ROUGHNESS

Q. Every time I shave, my neck gets red and a rash develops. I use a razor and a preshave lotion, but my skin still gets irritated. Is there anything I can do to minimize the damage?

—*D.L., Excelsior, Minn.*

A. You're experiencing what dermatologists call *pseudofolliculitis barbae.* That's "razor bumps" in plain English. These bumps can take the form of a rash, or they can look like little inflamed pimples under the chin and on the neck. They're caused when sharp, newly cut whiskers curl back around and reenter the skin. Although this condition is more common among black men, others are also afflicted by it.

The easiest solution is to grow a beard, since the coiled whiskers will spring back out of the skin once they are about half an inch long. If this isn't a viable option, the tips listed below, from Oakland, California, skin-care expert Kathryn Leverette, will help you get a clean shave without the bumps.

■ Soak your razor in alcohol for ten minutes before shaving.
■ Use a sudsing antibacterial soap or unscented shaving cream to lather up.
■ Shave only in the direction of hair growth.
■ Don't stretch the skin to shave closer. When the skin bounces back, the shaved hair will be trapped below the skin line.
■ After shaving, use a nonirritating, nonalcohol tonic.

HATLESS

Q. I used to wear a hat all the time, but recently stopped because several people told me that doing so would make me lose my hair. I miss my hats, but I'd miss my hair more.

—N.W., Boston, Mass.

A. Heredity, not headgear, determines whether a man will go bald. Wearing tight-fitting football helmets or welding masks day after day can speed hair loss in men prone to baldness by decreasing the blood supply to the hair follicles, causing them to die prematurely, says Dr. John Romano. But the average hat is unlikely to pose any threat to your locks, no matter what your genetic propensity.

FEAR OF SPEAKING

Q. I dread having to speak before a crowd, yet my job demands that I occasionally give presentations to groups of up to 35 people. How can I overcome my fear and become a better speaker?

—K.B., Walla Walla, Wash.

A. "Most of the best speakers still get a little nervous even though they've given hundreds or thousands of talks," says Al Walker, president of the National Speakers Association. "But if you're properly prepared, that nervous energy can be the difference between a flat speech and a lively one."

That said, good speakers do use certain tricks that allow them to shine when the spotlight is on. To harness your adrenaline and improve your speaking ability, try the following:

Memorize both ends. By carefully planning an opening and a closing, you'll cut down on your prespeech anxiety, and you also won't have to spend the last third of your talk worrying about how you're going to wind things up.

Make allies. During your speech, make eye contact with various individuals in the room for a few seconds, enough to elicit a facial expression. People who acknowledge you with a smile or a nod are usually on your side, and you should turn back to them periodically throughout your speech. "Work with the people who show approval and let them win the others over," says Walker.

Have extra information. Speakers typically tend to talk much faster when they're actually giving a speech than when they are just practicing. It's a good rule of thumb to go in with twice as much information as you need so you don't run out of things to say 10 minutes into a 15-minute speech.

Practice. Consider joining a local chapter of Toastmasters International (714-858-8255), a nonprofit organization devoted to teaching the art of public speaking. Chapter members get together weekly to take turns at the podium. Or, consider taking a public-speaking class or hiring a speech coach.

PREWORKOUT NIBBLES

Q. I've heard numerous theories on whether or not it's a good idea to eat before a workout. One claimed that food consumed immediately prior to a workout is not important because the energy for exercise comes from food consumed 10 to 12 hours earlier. Another stated that a small preworkout meal is essential to maximize performance. What's the best nutritional strategy to help me get the most out of my workouts?

—*M.H., Williston, Vt.*

A. Energy for exercise comes from foods eaten anytime during the 48 hours prior to exercise, *including* those consumed immediately before the workout. When deciding whether or not to eat before a workout, you have to consider what type of exercise you will be doing, how long it will last and when you ate your last meal, says Liz Applegate, Ph.D., author of *Power Foods*. Aerobic exercise such as running or cycling tends to last longer and burn more calories than weight workouts, and for these you may find it especially beneficial to consume a snack of 200 to 300 calories 15 to 30 minutes before starting. Ideal choices include high-carbohydrate foods like fruit, fig bars, energy bars or sports drinks. All of these can make it into the bloodstream within 15 minutes.

A snack also makes good sense before any kind of exercise if you haven't eaten for more than four hours. "To be at your best, never go into a workout without eating if you feel you have an empty stomach or are light-headed," suggests Dr. Applegate. "But avoid eating a large meal or snack because it will divert blood from working muscles into the digestive tract. Also, foods high in protein and fat are much slower to digest than carbohydrates."

For endurance workouts lasting well over an hour, it is best to eat a little before the workout and resupply at regular intervals while you exercise.

TOO FEW Z'S

Q. As a paramedic in a large city, I'm often forced to work long hours. There are lots of nights when I get only three or four hours of sleep. Is this doing long-term damage to my body? If so, is there anything I can do to minimize the ill effects?

—*S.C., San Jose, Calif.*

A. Getting by on three or four hours of sleep once a week won't hurt you. You may feel awful the next day, but you can probably handle it. Catch up by getting to bed earlier the next night or by grabbing a quick nap whenever you can.

If you're losing more than ten hours of sleep a week, however, you could be building up a sleep deficit that's harder to restore. According to Terry Phillips, Ph.D., D.Sc., an immunologist at George Washington University Medical Center, your immune system plummets and mental skills decline when you routinely short your body of sleep.

If that's the case, the best thing you can do is try to catch up, though doing so is not easy. Depending on the size of your sleep deficit, recovering can take a month or more. Considering the demands of your job, you may have to force yourself to go to bed earlier on those nights when you can, even if there are things you'd rather be doing. While you work on paying back your sleep debt, boost your day-to-day energy level with the following tips.

■ Go for a high-protein lunch. Studies show that men whose noontime meal is high in protein have much more afternoon gusto than those who go for carbohydrates. Healthy high-protein choices include tuna, poultry and low-fat yogurt.

■ Cover your bases. Take a daily multivitamin supplement to ensure that your body's getting the supplies it needs. Vitamin deficiency will only enhance your dragged-out feeling.

■ Get some exercise, but not too much. A brisk ten-minute walk will increase blood circulation, sending more oxygen to the muscles and to the brain. Studies show that even brief exercise boosts energy levels for up to two hours.

TOUGH TUMMY

Q. I've been doing a lot of stomach crunches to prepare for a physical-fitness test. In the process I've gained an inch of muscle on my stomach, and now all my pants are snug. How can I strengthen my abdominal muscles without building a "muscle potbelly"?

—T.H., San Diego, Calif.

A. Although it's not impossible to gain an inch of muscle around your midsection over the course of several months, it's our guess that your new belly is made more of fat than muscle. For one thing, stomach crunches tend to isolate the upper abdominals and ignore the lower, making it very unlikely that your routine would put that much bulk around your waistline. In addition, although abdominal muscles do increase in size with use, they typically push organs inward, not out, producing a tight, washboard look, says Charles Kuntzleman, Ed.D., associate professor of physical education at the University of Michigan.

If you disagree, try the pinch-poke test. If you can pinch more than an inch of skin off your stomach or your index finger sinks into your belly past its first joint, the problem is fat, not muscle. Many men who switch from an aerobic-type fitness program to a strength- or calisthenics-based routine gain a few pounds until they adjust their diets for the fact that they're burning fewer calories, even though they're exercising just as long. To tighten your lower abdomen, Dr. Kuntzleman suggests curlbacks: Sit on the floor with your knees up and your arms crossed over your chest. Moving backward, lower your upper body until you feel a "tug." Hold this position for three to five seconds; return to original position. Do 10 to 15 repetitions per day.

TESTY TESTICLES

Q. For several months I've had an ache in my testicles. Sometimes the pain is severe, sometimes mild, and other times there's no pain at all. I checked for any lumps that might have signaled cancer, but fortunately I didn't find any. What could be causing my pain, and is there anything I can do to make it go away?

—*E.L., Kansas City, Kans.*

A. Cancerous lumps in the testicles rarely produce any pain. (That's actually one of the reasons men need to examine themselves regularly.) Take your problem to a urologist to see if the cause might be an infection. If so, he'll probably put you on an antibiotic, which should clear up the problem in less than three weeks.

If you don't have an infection, your pain may be the result of a hernia or partially obstructed epididymis, the narrow, curly tube that coils around the outside of your testicles. Another possibility is *intermittent torsion*, a condition in which the testicles swivel on themselves, cutting off blood supply to the area. As the name implies, the torsion can subside only to recur; therefore it is easier to diagnose while you're still experiencing pain. In some rare cases, testicular pain has no discernible origin. Such cases typically resolve themselves over time, but to be safe, see a doctor.

ONE O'CLOCK SHADOW

Q. I've heard of a five o'clock shadow, but mine is usually visible by 1:00 P.M. I've used electric and disposable razors, but I just can't seem to get close enough to keep my whiskers down all day. What am I doing wrong?

—*D.M., West Norriton, Pa.*

A. The speed of beard growth varies little, but some men like you have a very full, dark beard that makes its presence known even when it's short. The only practical thing you can do to minimize your afternoon shadow is to give yourself an ultraclose shave every morning, says Dr. John Romano. To do this without irritating your skin, start by lathering your beard with soap and warm water to soften the whiskers. Without rinsing off the soap, spread on a shaving gel, and using a sharp razor, shave in the direction of hair growth.

Keep a rechargeable electric razor in your desk drawer at work and use it for afternoon touch-ups.

MORNING EYES

Q. Many mornings when I wake up, my eyes are red and swollen. Although the problem usually clears itself up within an hour or two, it does get annoying. Is there anything I can do to see my way out of this?

—*T.C., Merritt Island, Fla.*

A. Pack those bags, pal. Your problem, the result of fluid collecting around your eyes, is probably caused by sleeping on your stomach or without a pillow. This puts your head level with or below your heart and allows fluid to accumulate around your eyes. "Anytime blood has to move uphill to get back to the heart, there is an increased tendency for swelling," says ophthalmologist Thomas O. Burkholder, M.D.

The swelling dissipates when you get out of bed because gravity pulls the fluid back toward the heart. You can avoid, or minimize, that morning-zombie look by sleeping on your back or side and propping your head up with a pillow or two.

Excessive fatigue and alcohol can make the swelling worse, since they dilate the tiny vessels around the eyes and let fluid build up. If your swelling is more severe at certain times of the year, you may be suffering from allergies.

BUILDING TRUST

Q. I'm 35 and have recently begun dating a 33-year-old divorced woman who has three kids. I have a great relationship with two of her kids, but the oldest, a ten-year-old boy, won't have anything to do with me. How can I win him over?

—T.S., Lancaster, Pa.

A. "Chances are, he doesn't have anything against you personally; he's just protecting his territory," says Bruce Fisher, Ed.D., author of *Rebuilding: When Your Relationship Ends.* He says that after a divorce, the oldest boy often assumes the role of the man of the family and feels he has to protect his mother from being hurt again.

To show him you're not just there to see his mother, Dr. Fisher suggests you set aside a few days a month to do something with him and his siblings. It can be a hike, a fishing trip, a baseball game or anything they enjoy. It's best if their mother doesn't come along. If she does, the boy is more likely to slip back into his role of protector.

If things don't start to improve within a few months, and you're serious about your relationship, consider some family counseling. You can get a list of qualified family therapists in your area by calling the American Association for Marriage and Family Therapy at (800) 374-2638.

Index

A

Abdomen. *See also* Stomach
  pain in, 69–70, 173
  strengthening muscles
    of, 190–93, 242–44,
    285–86
Achilles tendon, 175, 221
Acquired Immune
  Deficiency Syndrome
  (AIDS), testing for, 178,
  180
Adrenaline, 137
Aerobic exercise. *See also*
  Exercise
  benefits of, 184–85, 242
  to keep mentally sharp,
    10
  to lower blood pres-
    sure, 184
Aggression, 79–85
  anger and, 86–87
  release of, 81–82

  repression vs. suppres-
    sion, 83–84
Aging, 1–10
  attitudes about, 10
  effects of sun and, 6–7
  slowing, 1–10
AIDS, testing for, 178, 180
Alcohol
  and cancer, 161
  decreasing intake of,
    63–68
  in moderation, 9, 36,
    63–68
  risks, 166
  tips for safe drinking,
    63–68
  and weight loss,
    247–48
Anger, 82–85, 86–87
Angina, 173
Ankle pain, 232–33